# THE EMERGING FIELD OF SOCIOBIBLIOGRAPHY

**RECENT TITLES IN CONTRIBUTIONS IN LIBRARIANSHIP AND INFORMATION SCIENCE**

SERIES EDITOR: *Paul Wasserman*

Subject Retrieval in the Seventies: New Directions. An International Symposium
*Hans (Hanan) Wellisch and Thomas D. Wilson, Editors*

Quantitative Methods in Librarianship: Standards, Research, Management
*Irene Braden Hoadley and Alice S. Clark, Editors*

Public Relations for Libraries: Essays in Communications Techniques
*Allan Angoff, Editor*

Human Memory and Knowledge: A Systems Approach
*Glynn Harmon*

Libraries in the Political Scene: Georg Leyh and German Librarianship, 1933-1953
*Marta L. Dosa*

Information Retrieval and Documentation in Chemistry
*Charles H. Davis and James E. Rush*

Illustrative Computer Programming for Libraries: Selected Examples for Information Specialists
*Charles H. Davis*

University Science and Engineering Libraries: Their Operation, Collections, and Facilities
*Ellis Mount*

Participative Management in Academic Libraries
*Maurice P. Marchant*

Libraries As Communication Systems
*J. M. Orr*

A Community Elite and the Public Library: The Uses of Information in Leadership
*Pauline Wilson*

# THE EMERGING FIELD OF SOCIOBIBLIOGRAPHY

## *The Collected Essays of Ilse Bry*

Edited and Compiled by
LOIS AFFLERBACH and
MARGA FRANCK

Contributions in Librarianship and
Information Science, Number 19

GREENWOOD PRESS
Westport, Connecticut • London, England

**Library of Congress Cataloging in Publication Data**

Bry, Ilse.
The emerging field of sociobibliography.

(Contributions in librarianship and information science ; no. 19)
Includes index.
1. Psychology–Bibliography. 2. Psychiatry–Bibliography. 3. Social sciences–Bibliography.
I. Title.
Z7201.A2B79 [BF38] 010'.28 76-28644
ISBN 0-8371-9289-7



Library of Congress Catalog Card Number: 76-28644
ISBN: 0-8371-9289-7

First published in 1977

Greenwood Press, Inc.
51 Riverside Avenue, Westport, Connecticut 06880

Printed in the United States of America

# Contents

# Foreword

The publication of these essays, which are attributed to Dr. Ilse Bry by her former colleagues on the Editorial Committee of the *Mental Health Book Review Index,* is a felicitous event in the history of contemporary librarianship. Those who haven't previously known her work will be afforded deep insights into a brilliant and creative intelligence. Others, who have followed the editorials, the original form in which most of the essays appeared, in the *Mental Health Book Review Index,* will be reminded of Dr. Bry's encyclopedic knowledge of the literature of the behavioral sciences, but above all of her ability to identify new fields and trends, to interpret and explain hitherto unnoticed subject relationships, and to apply an organizing principle to the vast flow of this literature.

A chronological review of the essays gives evidence of a steady progression in the depth and range of her thinking which would culminate in the concept of sociobibliography, a professional contribution of the first magnitude. In "Is Bibliographic Standardization Possible?" some fundamental concerns are expressed about the feasibility of the cataloging in source experiment as a possible means of standardizing bibliographic usage. Succeeding essays examine the problems of organizing scientific knowledge, discuss methods of identifying the significant literature of a field, and note a variety of ways to utilize book reviews for these purposes.

The essays published from 1963 onwards reflect new concerns about the rapidly changing environment in which scientific literature is being produced and contain some of Bry's most sensitive and scholarly contributions. "Changes in the Concept of 'Scientific Literature' " points to the implications of a new "shift of emphasis which has put *information,* not *literature,* in the center of attention." The indiscriminate use of the computer is criticized in "Bibliographical Challenges in the Age of the Computer." Four essays published between 1965 and 1969 explore the problem of finding an organizing principle for the behavioral sciences, show relationships between the human sciences and the humanities, suggest how bibliography can contribute to a better understanding and treatment of the history of the behavioral sciences, and offer a critical analysis of the growth patterns of the literature.

In 1970 Dr. Bry introduced in a formal sense the seminal concept of sociobibliography in: "Lectureships in the Behavioral Sciences–An Introduction to Sociobibliography." She suggested the intriguing possibilities of a series of studies of lectures in the behavioral sciences. One of these studies would apply the methodology of social research to identify lectureships as cultural phenomena.

In "The Emerging Field of Sociobibliography: Reassessment and Reorientation of Access to Knowledge in the Social Sciences," the last essay, sociobibliography emerges fully as a scientific approach to bibliography. The interrelationships between the social sciences and bibliography are explored in detail. Bibliographical and scientific methods are combined to identify the social and cultural as well as scientific significance of new knowledge. Problems of access to the literature of the social sciences are made more susceptible of solutions by applying the proposed methodology. Finally, principles of sociobibliography are laid down which appear to open the way to new interpretations of the history of ideas and social history, and to suggest how uncontrollable growth of scientific publication can be avoided.

This collection of scholarly essays is a distinguished, original contribution to librarianship and to a better understanding of the evolving behavioral sciences.

Morris A. Gelfand
Professor and Chairman,
Department of Library Science
Queens College

# *Preface*

The plan to publish this collection of essays originated several years before Dr. Bry's terminal illness. She herself described the book's purpose in a letter to the editor of the series Contributions in Librarianship and Information Science: "In various recent papers I have introduced and illustrated the concept of sociobibliography. I should like to make that the focus of the book . . . . The crux of the matter, as I see it, is that the literature of the behavioral sciences is submerged in the bibliographic organization with which we must work. What brings this literature to light in its own right are the methods developed in sociobibliography."

All fourteen essays appeared originally as editorials in the *Mental Health Book Review Index,** an annual list of books selected and reviewed by specialists and organized as a bibliography by librarians. The 255 journals from which the book reviews were taken relate to the behavioral sciences and the field of mental health. A number of essays were edited by Dr. Bry for publication in an extended and documented version in various behavioral science or library journals. Others were prepared for the present volume by its editors in order to ensure a consistent bibliographic format.

Lois Afflerbach
Marga Franck

*The editorials were all written in collaboration, but her co-author, Lois Afflerbach, is the first to emphasize the primacy of Dr. Bry's contribution to each of them.

# *Introduction*

Trained primarily as a philosopher and as a librarian, Ilse Bry made noteworthy and lasting contributions to the field of mental health. She was a scientist as well as a librarian: she obtained a master's degree in psychology at Columbia University, and in the process she learned a good deal about the research techniques of psychology and developed a sense of identity as a psychologist, reflected in her lasting membership in the American Psychological Association. She not only attended many conventions, but with characteristic thoroughness and conscientiousness participated more actively than most in the governance of this and other scientific organizations to which she belonged (such as the American Association for the Advancement of Science, the Council of Biology Editors, and the Federation of American Scientists). Even while she held an appointment as research assistant in the Research Center for Mental Health, New York University, she was far too modest ever to present herself as a member of the group she called "subject-matter experts in the behavioral sciences."

Three kinds of contributions she made come readily to mind. The first is conceptual: her scholarly treatment of the problem of defining the behavioral sciences. Her broad intellectual perspective came from her experience and training in wrestling with the problem of conceptually organizing the entire sweep of human intellectual activity. Everyone concedes that the day of the "Renaissance man," who knew something about all important branches of learning, has gone; yet the custodians of man's heritage of written knowledge must still face the problem of how to organize that enormous corpus of diverse achievement. For if books are to be acquired, stored, retrieved, and made available for use by scholars, they must be rationally classified. Armed as she was with a knowledge of the various systems that had been proposed and used, in addition to the now ubiquitous Library of Congress classification, Dr. Bry knew in intimate detail the problems faced by any emerging new grouping of disciplines or by those who wanted to identify its literature.

Her experience in two important libraries in the field of mental health (Abraham A. Brill Library of the New York Psychoanalytic Institute, and the large neuropsychiatric collection of the New York University-Bellevue Medical Center), confirmed her theory that the relevant discipline basic to mental health was far broader than psychiatry and/or psychology. The intellectual substrate of the mental health practitioner was nothing less than the emerging new cluster of *behavioral sciences.* Dr. Bry devoted herself to the *Mental Health Book Review Index* over so many years and with such extraordinary persistence and scholarly effectiveness because she saw it as something much more than simply a handy reference tool. It was, first of all, a device for helping to define the field of the behavioral sciences themselves. Several of the papers reprinted here describe how she used it to attain both operational and conceptual definitions of what was for all its modishness a rather evanescent term.

A second kind of contribution–methodological–emerged from her successful effort to make the *Index* a research tool. What began as the systematic checking of essential information about every book listed in the publication ended up as a collection of data in which she saw many kinds of usefulness. In a sense, a science *is* its cumulative literature; bibliographic methods therefore can be much more than just a means for locating information, for as Dr. Bry showed they turn up unexpectedly rich data about the ways scientists define, control, and shape the total body of information they call their discipline. Such social institutions as the Festschrift, the memorial lecture series, and the special topic symposium lead to distinctive types of publication which may be used to index the underlying value judgments, forms of social control, or the like.

Such was the purview of *sociobibliography,* a term she introduced in her invited contribution to the *International Encyclopedia of the Social Sciences.* That invitation was, incidentally, the high point of Dr. Bry's international recognition as the outstanding authority on the bibliography of the behavioral sciences, and the breadth of vision embodied in her article indicates the appropriateness of that reputation. Unfortunately, Dr. Bry did not live to carry out most of the substantive applications of research methods that she had envisaged, but the present record of her methodological contributions may well inspire and assist other workers in such fields as the history of science and the sociology of knowledge.

Third, she completed and published some applications of bibliographic method to the history of science. I have in mind particularly the valuable and frequently cited paper she wrote in collaboration with Alfred Rifkin on several controversial aspects of Freud's career, which has done a great deal to deflate several myths and to explain some previously mysterious points in his life and career.[1]

These are the principal contributions that to me stand out among many lesser ones. But this book as a whole can be warmly recommended to "subject-matter experts"—or, more modestly, practitioners—in the mental health field and to behavioral scientists generally for its many valuable conceptual insights, original contributions to method, and nuggets of information about the history of ideas. This collection of a gifted scientist's work is an exemplary model of selfless, thorough scholarship of a quality all too rarely seen today.

Robert R. Holt
Research Center for Mental Health
New York University

## NOTE

1. Rifkin, Alfred H., and Ilse Bry. "Freud and the History of Ideas: Primary Sources, 1886-1910." (*In Science and Psychoanalysis,* vol. 5, (New York, Grune & Stratton, 1962), pp. 6-36.)

# THE EMERGING FIELD OF SOCIOBIBLIOGRAPHY

# ESSAY 1

## *Is Bibliographic Standardization Possible?*

*With an introduction by Esther J. Piercy and comments by George Piternick*

Originally published as Editorial in *Mental Health Book Review Index,* vol. 4, no. 2 (whole no. 8), July 1959. Reprinted by permission of the American Library Association from *Library Resources and Technical Services,* Winter 1960, pp. 67-70.

Without attempting to document the statement, it is probably safe to say that the goal of standardizing bibliographic usage is as old as scholarship itself.

Recently the concept has returned to prominent discussion because of the Cataloging in Source experiment. One of the great accomplishments foreseen for that service would be the printing of a catalog entry within each book, thus providing an always-accessible entry available to cataloger and bibliographer alike. Thus, if catalogers, reference workers, bibliographers, scholars, writers, publishers, book dealers, and all others concerned with handling, citing, or discussing books could be persuaded to follow the same entry, the means would be at hand. Aside from the feasibility of the CIS service, would it, if available, be so used? Can we get the often-expressed variance in library and bibliographic purpose compromised? Is there a possible meeting ground of purpose and practice? If so, who will be served and who will suffer? These are questions requiring discussion and airing.

One such discussion recently appeared in print and was called to our attention by Lucile M. Morsch, Deputy Chief Assistant Librarian, Library of Congress. The July, 1959, (v. 4, no. 2) issue of the *Mental Health Book Review Index* carried an editorial, parts of which read:

"Book reviews exert an influence not only as a medium of selection and criticism, but also, more subtly, through bibliographic entries. These entail decisions of the reviewers or editors regarding authorship of the books reviewed. In the mental health sciences, the specialists, who often review the same books, appear to agree on the principle of attributing authorship. They follow—and thereby sustain—a tradition that is admittedly no longer fully applicable to many books published today. Whether intended or not, their entries single out the senior author for explicit credit. Even when additional authors are included in the original citation, the longer the list of names, the sooner will it give way to the briefer *et al.*

"To a degree, this same usage prevails in libraries and library-oriented bibliographies. When books of complicated origin were still relatively rare, however, librarians introduced the concept of corporate author entry, to be used for works published in the name or by the authority of corporate bodies. They then linked the new with the old system by adding an entry under the appropriate personal name. Today the monographic literature as a whole has become far more complex. For instance, books with multiple authors are also apt to have multiple sponsors. Just as the first-named individual need no longer literally be the 'senior' author, but may take his place in alphabetical order rather than according to academic rank, so the listing of several sponsoring groups need not imply that any one of them has a particular claim to corporate authorship.

"These developments have strained the sense and use of both bibliographic traditions, and the gap between them has widened. Information deemed essential by librarians for identifying the book is often ignored by reviewers, or relegated to the descriptive part of the review, where it is lost for the citation. Conversely, recent library practice tends to omit names of individuals from the catalog, when the book is clearly based on a collective effort. As a result, it is often hard to recognize the same book under two almost completely different bibliographic guises.

"This issue of the *Mental Health Book Review Index* contains more than the usual number of examples illustrating this problem. We should like, therefore, to point out the main discrepancies. Specialists conceive of an author as a person, and only when no person is indicated as author, will they accept corporate authorship. This does not mean that the author must have written the book. Author status can be conferred upon editor, compiler, committee chairman, an authority signing the preface, the participants in a discussion, and the nameless, yet still personalized 'Various authors.' In current library practice, catalogs contain as author entries an abundance of carefully verified official names. These may be the names of conferences, of their sponsors or places of meeting, or, intermingled with well-known institutions and associations, the quite unfamiliar names of minor agencies and ad hoc committees. Works issued repeatedly, such as annual reviews, are recorded under their title; the title of a periodical from which articles were chosen for republication in book form, is also preferred over the editor's name; and in posthumous publications, the original writer remains the author, no matter how much the living compiler contributed in editing unpublished essays, letters, or notes.

"The divergent usage in bibliography can be explained by the difference in professional responsibilities. The person submitting the book to the scientific community ranks as author in its channels of communication, even when the book appears under official auspices. In library records that personal identity takes second place, and may even be lost, in favor of the more lasting, institutionalized, impersonal designation of authorship. Each approach is guided by a long-term view. The scientific community, which creates the history of ideas, identifies a name with a school of thought and often chooses the men who made a notable contribution as spokesmen for new developments. Those concerned with the continuity, structure, and permanent use of the literature, on the other hand, look for the organized authority behind the book that will outlast the individual and perhaps sponsor similar efforts. Attempts to impose the concepts of one group upon the practice of the other seem neither desirable nor likely to succeed.

"The *Mental Health Book Review Index* integrates the bibliographic interpretations of librarians and specialists. In principle, we follow the form of authorship accepted by the Library of Congress and printed in the *National Union Catalog,* the form in which books appear in the catalogs of most libraries in this country and in a growing number of libraries abroad. In giving additional bibliographic information, we include names and details which will be useful to specialists and librarians in the field of mental health. And in our cross-references, we connect the variations of bibliographic entry, usually the form prevailing in the reviews, with the form adopted in the interest of library cooperation."

Some attempt has been made to encourage more discussion on the subject. From George Piternick, Library Administrative Analyst of the University of California, Berkeley, comes some pertinent comment. Although it is main entry with which we are primarily concerned, his remarks are necessary to the background of the discussion. He says:

"It should be emphasized that most bibliographical entry of the type dealt with is single entry, whereas library catalog entry is multiple, and in this fact lies the basis for some reasonable compromise of objective and methods between the two camps. Basically, all that is desired is that people going from a bibliographical citation of a book to a library catalog will find information on whether or not the library possesses that book. It is desirable that this information be produced at the first step, but it is not essential; a cross-reference to a library entry for the book is adequate if not optimal. Neither is it necessary that the catalog user find a main entry card under the bibliographical citation with which he is armed; an added entry will suffice. What is intolerable is a blank, when the library actually has the book.

"Standardization of *main* entry among bibliographer and library catalogers does not seem feasible in view of the varying objectives of the two crafts, as pointed out by the authors. There seems no compelling reason, however, why there should not be a common entry between the single entry chosen by the bibliographer and the group of entries selected by the catalogers. This degree of standardization is both desirable and feasible, and, in fact, does exist in the majority of cases. To reduce the number of blind leads from citation to catalog, however, both camps must make adjustments.

"1. Bibliographers should make concerted effort to see that the personal name selected for entry when more than one is available should be the one most relevant to the concept of authorship, i.e., author over compiler, compiler over editor, editor over chairman of sponsoring group, etc. When personal entries are not available, the bibliographer should choose the corporate entry most relevant, i.e., corporate body producing a work over corporate body to which the work is addressed, etc.

"2. Catalogers and catalog codes should be cautious in continuing and extending the practice of reducing the number of added entries, especially personal added entries, and especially for works given corporate main entry. Certainly no work given corporate main entry, but including prominent display of a person or persons responsible for the preparation of the work, should be cataloged without providing added entry for the person most emphatically listed, as well as for title, if distinctive."

# ESSAY 2

## *The Behavioral Sciences and Mental Health in Relation to the Organization of Knowledge, the Organization of Science, and Bibliography*

Originally published as Editorial in *Mental Health Book Review Index,* vol. 5, no. 1 (whole no. 9), January 1960. Reprinted from the *A.M.A. Archives of General Psychiatry,* vol. 2, June 1960, pp. 701-706. 

1. The concept *behavioral sciences* emerged in the late 'Forties, a time of rising interest in the scientific study of man. Scholars in many fields of specialization felt the need to unify knowledge contributed to the understanding of human behavior from nearly all parts of the scientific world. The group of scientists who coined the term and later launched the journal *Behavioral Science,* chose the word "behavioral" from the psychologist's vocabulary because it was applicable to biological and social studies and acceptable to scientists in these fields as well.

In the past ten years the "behavioral sciences" have, however, come to mean many different things, often depending on the meaning attached to the word "behavioral." It can have strictly methodological connotations, for instance, when referring to the observation of behavior in contrast to the study of inner experience. When the term "behavioral sciences" is used to designate certain social sciences, this often separates psychology from psychiatry and psychoanalysis. In such cases the behavioral sciences lose their significance as a focus for a bio-psycho-social orientation.

A composite of those interpretations of the term which agree on the scientific goal, man's understanding of himself, suggests a tentative definition of the *behavioral sciences* as a multidisciplinary pursuit of knowledge about behavior in its roots and manifestations, in man and animals, in individuals, groups, and cultures, and in all conditions, normal, exceptional, and pathological.

Behavioral scientists remain specialists in their respective fields, while striving to unify their diverse theories and concepts. Against a multidisciplinary background they often concentrate on specific areas of study, such as child development or aging. A thorough discussion of the behavioral sciences today would take the scientific advances of a whole century into account, in which psychology, psychiatry, and later psychoanalysis have played a pioneering role.

The lines between the behavioral sciences and individual disciplines are by no means clearly or firmly drawn. A field that contributes to the scientific study of behavior does not cease to be part of its original discipline. Nor does the process of unifying knowledge that deals with human behavior from different points of view confer a new status on any established field of specialization. The resulting situation is far more complex than the word "interdisciplinary" can convey. For instance, the behavioral sciences encompass the study of human communication as well as that of delinquent behavior. Yet the former continues to belong primarily to philology and the latter to criminology. These are embedded in a more deeply entrenched structure, now almost a thousand years old, where one is part of Philosophy, the other of Jurisprudence, which with Theology and Medicine formed the four faculties of the first medieval universities.

Many difficulties experienced in efforts to advance the behavioral sciences stem from their need to draw on fields of learning that may be organized under any of these four faculties in their present form. In many other now converging fields, scientists need to cross only disciplinary lines between subdivisions which earlier formed a whole. Those who are developing a science of behavior, however, must cross boundaries intended to separate, not to link the great realms of knowledge.

In our universities, for example, departments of psychology and of psychiatry are separate administrative units, conferring different academic degrees, and often physically miles apart, one being located on the main campus, the other in the medical school, which may even be in another city. Their literature and library resources are organized within the same framework that divided Philosophy from Medicine. This background creates a special problem for bibliographic and library services in "psychology–psychiatry," as the nucleus of the "behavioral sciences" is sometimes called.

Further underlying these difficulties is a conflict between the direction in which the behavioral sciences are moving and the perspective created by the traditional organization of knowledge. It has been a persistent concept that the totality of knowledge can be systematized in the image of a tree with its branches, or a classification scheme with divisions and subdivisions, allowing for future specialization, which will not involve the established system of the past. The organization of knowledge was initially a scheme of ideas. It is now more tangible than that because it is intimately related to the organization of science. The latter comprises all functions of the scientific community, its institutions of training and research, the organizations of scientists and scholars, their means of communication, and their joint scientific operations.

The pursuit of new knowledge may, however, lead to developments that had not been anticipated at all. Adaptations within the available organization of knowledge are being made continually, but from time to time a radical change becomes necessary. One of these epochal changes began in the seventeenth century. Then the rise of modern science opened fields of investigation which became superimposed upon the older structure, without displacing it.

The new organization of knowledge could not again, as in the Middle Ages, strike roots so deeply in our academic life, but it became the organizing force for another great development in the history of organized science and scholarship, on which our contemporary concept of a scientific community rests. First academies of science arose, among which the Royal Society of London with its *Philosophical Transactions* is still one of the best known. From these grew innumerable learned societies and organizations devoted to the advancement of more specific fields. Similarly, the first periodicals, such as the *Journal des Sçavans,* which extended communication among all scholars, were the forerunners of the host of specialized journals and bibliographies of our time.

Eventually, three major groupings of the many fields of specialization crystallized: the Natural Sciences, which explore the inanimate and animate universe in which man finds himself; the Social Sciences, concerned with the political, social, legal, and economic structure he has given to the world around him; and the Humanities, the study of man's lasting intellectual and artistic creations.

The behavioral sciences, which cut across the present counterparts of the medieval faculties, also have a direct interchange with fields assigned to any of these more recent divisions in the contemporary scheme of all knowledge.

2. In contrast to the behavioral sciences, which are confined within the scientific community, *mental health* has become a matter of activity for the community at large. There has been no more place for mental health than for the behavioral sciences on any existing map of the organization of knowledge. Thus in administrative arrangements, "mental health" has had to be allocated to one or another established area. The choice has varied from the social sciences, the life sciences, or psychology, to medicine, psychiatry, or public health.

The term "mental health," too, has assumed a variety of meanings. It has absorbed changing popular notions, such as "peace of mind" or "adjustment." At the same time, it has served as a synonym for mental hygiene and as a euphemism for mental illness. More recently, efforts have been made to reserve the concept of mental health for a standard of well-being and of human relations, regardless of the still unsettled question what such a standard should be. In a fifth meaning, associated with the governmental and nongovernmental programs internationally guided by the World Health Organization and the World Federation for Mental Health, the term has become the name for a field of endeavor, having the dynamics of a social movement and aimed at attaining the highest standards of mental health for all peoples and nations of the world.

In its scientific core, the field of mental health is based on knowledge evolved in the behavioral sciences. The field is broadened in another direction. It includes professional applications of this knowledge, for instance, when it is adapted to the specific professional training and tasks of teachers, social workers, nurses, ministers, and law enforcement officers. Furthermore, the mental health movement is vitally concerned with disseminating this knowledge in adaptations for lay use and understanding. It considers a wide range of problems, before and after they have become amenable to the methods of the behavioral sciences, and takes an active part in reform. For example, when findings of the behavioral sciences have an impact on legislation or otherwise lead to social action, the research findings as well as their application and influence, whether in the realm of science or society, would be within the range of the mental health movement.

*Mental Health* as a field, therefore, makes use of a core of knowledge, contributed by the behavioral sciences, and amplifies it with scientific, professional, and social ramifications and applications. It is in this sense that we interpret the name of the *Mental Health Book Review Index.*

3. The role of bibliographies and libraries in the organization of knowledge has been a traditional theme in the literature of library science and documentation, now often treated with a sense of urgency. The place of the behavioral sciences in contemporary bibliography, specifically, does not yet seem to have attracted the attention it deserves.

During the nineteenth century, the scientific community took a new step in the organization of science, by creating systematic, specialized bibliographies. These were designed to represent, in a condensed, continuous record, the total achievement of a discipline within the context of its allied fields. Those members of the scientific community who served it in an editorial function were already responsible for deciding which manuscripts merited publication. Selection among publications by the editors of bibliographies appeared as a more radical step. It implicitly sanctioned a new standard of scholarship in science, since it had been the mark of scholarship to rely only on primary sources. The new conception, somewhat comparable to the delegation of judicial functions in the civic community, secured the support of learned societies, the collaboration of scientists and scholars, and, in the leading roles, the dedication of eminent men.

The various bibliographic instruments, of which the German *Zentralblätter* were outstanding examples, became a more important means of international scientific communication until the First World War. They could gain this importance because the organization of science, evolved over the preceding two hundred years, had been sufficiently consolidated to support an intervening stage between the individual scholar and the, for him, overwhelming mass of primary publications. The editors, themselves distinguished scholars in their fields, were able to utilize for their bibliographies the scientific organization that entered, for instance, into the sponsoring and editing of subject journals or the issuing of society transactions. Thus a first measure of merit and pertinence was already provided, when the bibliographers gathered together a body of literature representative of the progress in their field and comprehensive enough to inform individual scientists of research pertinent to their own. With an international network of scientific cooperation, the editors could then subject this literature to the desired degree of analysis, condensation, and assessment, rearrange the bibliographic items in suitable classifications, and make them available for reference through name and subject indexes.

This indirect use of the organization of science for bibliographic purposes was naturally most productive in the well-established disciplines, particularly in those rich in primary publications, such as medicine. Some early psychological bibliographies which, like the *Psychological Index,* were initiated late in the nineteenth century, show the extraordinary integrative effort that had to be made in a field just beginning to be organized, in order to match the excellence of the bibliographies in older fields. Psychologists as bibliographers, therefore, contributed greatly to the organization of their science by identifying pertinent work, no matter under which disciplinary auspices it was published.

In the twentieth century, the organization of science had progressed so far that it became possible to build upon it still more comprehensive bibliographic and scientific information services for various important areas. Abstracting and indexing services were increasingly staffed with professional personnel and issued under large administrative auspices, partly governmental, sometimes international. As a rule, the scientific community concentrated its efforts on reviewing and evaluating advances. An appraisal of the place the behavioral sciences hold in contemporary bibliography must take this relationship between the organization of science and various modes of bibliographic control into account.

The situation varies, for example, with respect to psychiatry and psychology. Both began in the second half of the nineteenth century to reach a growing independence from their parent disciplines. Today, the periodical literature identified with psychiatry, which includes part of psychoanalysis and abnormal psychology, is treated on equal terms with that of other recognized medical specialties. It is, therefore, covered in the comprehensive, international bibliographic services in medicine, supplemented by others originating in neighboring fields, such as biology, chemistry, and psychology. Specialists in psychiatry and psychoanalysis add to this their selective, annual reviews of progress.

The growth of the field of psychology has given rise to a body of literature published under the auspices of psychology as an independent discipline. This has made the task of bibliographic synthesis less demanding than it was, when the material was scattered and only a few psychological journals existed. Psychologists are, however, still themselves conducting nearly all their bibliographic services, with a view to selecting contributions to psychology; to that end, they include books as well as articles and continue to search nonpsychological publications. An adjustment to the growing volume of the international literature has been made, not by expanding administrative provisions, but by constricting the boundaries of bibliographic content.

One more development should be mentioned. That is the automation being promoted by the documentation movement. From different points of view, documentalists and behavioral scientists share an interest in computer and electronic systems development, including research on information processing. Any applications of research results from these fields to the problems of identifying, unifying, and analyzing the literature of the behavioral sciences are, however, entirely remote. The human effort that must precede the proper use of mechanical devices still needs to be made. The creators of these machines, which extend man's intellectual power beyond the limits of his speed and endurance, have always cautioned that no new Minerva will ever spring from a Jovian electronic brain.

The bibliographer's and librarian's scholarly function does not change with his instruments. In fulfilling this function, the librarian observes new phases in the organization of knowledge and of science, develops services for the further advancement of knowledge, and, in addition to unifying the literature of the field he serves, he ensures its continuity.

To study ways of applying the librarian's scholarly function to the behavioral sciences and mental health is one of the tasks we have set for ourselves in the *Mental Health Book Review Index.* Thus over the past five years we have been trying to trace with bibliographic means how this sector of the scientific community is advancing its scientific organization, through conferences and symposia, newly founded academies and their proceedings, new multidisciplinary societies and institutes, an array of similarly new or reoriented journals, and, perhaps most effectively under conditions of such diversity, through the creation of a monographic literature with a network of cross-disciplinary evaluation.

If scholarly bibliography is to keep pace with this extensive and fast-moving frontier of contemporary knowledge, it will be necessary to search for an equally flexible bibliographic method. At this stage, it should unify a multidisciplinary content and reveal new areas of concentration, without obliterating the still meaningful disciplinary origins.

The *Mental Health Book Review Index* is a step toward a needed methodical inquiry. In this sense, it is offered as a service to the scientific community and to all who, from whatever point of view, share this interest.

# ESSAY 3

## *In Search of a Method of Identifying the Significant Monographic Literature of the Behavioral Sciences*

Originally published as Editorial in *Mental Health Book Review Index,* vol. 5, no. 2 (whole no. 10), July 1960.

In the *Mental Health Book Review Index,* 1956-1960, we have applied an exploratory technique, from which we are now able to derive a more selective bibliographic method.

During the past five years we have (1) evolved a list of journals in the English language which relate to the behavioral sciences and contribute to the evaluation of books; (2) put on file the references to all book reviews that appear in these journals, beginning with the volumes current in January, 1955; (3) listed in the *Mental Health Book Review Index* those books for which we could cite three or more reviews; and (4) continued to publish review references in groups of three or more for books previously listed.

The journals selected, at first most of them in the core subjects, psychology, psychiatry, and psychoanalysis and published in the United States, have grown in number from 50 to 132. Besides adding newly published journals, we have gradually included more journals from related fields and from the following countries: Australia, Canada, Great Britain, India, Japan, and South Africa. We now have identified about 7,350 books and pamphlets, of which 1,753 have been listed in the *Mental Health Book Review Index,* 1956-1960, together with almost 8,500 citations of reviews.

Our data have thus become substantial enough to show distinct and sometimes surprisingly stable patterns. For example, while we have almost tripled the number of journals indexed, we have consistently found that slightly less than one fourth of all the books reviewed received three or more reviews. The *Index* has demonstrated, however, that the number of reviews is no measure of the value of the book. If a book is widely reviewed, this may be due, among other reasons, to a timely topic, an element of prestige or challenge, an ample supply of review copies, or even a wish to register protest, shared by many reviewers. Nevertheless, since many more books are being offered for review to the scientific community than are accepted by it, those that receive a great deal of attention become significant, if not individually, then as components of an evolving literature.

Furthermore, we now know that scholarly exchanges of reactions to a book can last as long as five years. In this issue, we list for the sixth time Meehl's *Clinical Versus Statistical Prediction* (1954), and for the fourth time *Social Class and Mental Illness,* by Hollingshead and Redlich (1958). For each of these books we have so far cited 26 reviews, not counting comment and controversy. The assumption that reviews, to be most useful, must quickly follow publication, might be challenged by tracing critical opinion which has taken years to crystallize.

The number of books that enter into this assessment by the scientific community, the number of reviews that come out of it, and the duration of the process are background data which can now guide us in planning the next step. We seek an objective method of selecting books in the behavioral sciences and mental health, and a new way of organizing this literature.

In an earlier editorial we defined the *behavioral sciences* in part as a multidisciplinary pursuit of knowledge about behavior in all conditions, normal, exceptional, and pathological, and *mental health* as a field which amplifies the available knowledge with scientific, professional, and social ramifications and applications. Both terms are currently used to refer to multidisciplinary work, but neither is found in bibliographic usage. In handling the literature, specialists and librarians continue to use the names of the contributing disciplines, in particular psychology, psychiatry, or psychoanalysis, for the subjects in their narrower sense as well as for the behavioral sciences and mental health. No bibliography presents a record of major interests and achievements in the behavioral sciences, which the specialists and the public could recognize as such. Moreover, the behavioral sciences cannot be seen as an entity advancing side by side with other sciences, where scientific publications are collectively recorded, for instance, in general and subject bibliographies, in publication statistics, in libraries, or even in the media of the book trade. It is unpredictable how this literature will be dispersed, and where it will be absorbed in the categories now used.

The *Mental Health Book Review Index* is concerned with this difficulty. The books listed in its first ten issues are neither a selection of outstanding contributions nor a representative sample of the recent behavioral-science literature. We should like to take them for what they are, namely, the books on which the specialists in these fields, for whatever reasons, chose to concentrate their critical attention during the middle and late 'Fifties. These books tend to fall into three categories: (a) those reviewed from the standpoint of a single discipline or profession; (b) those reviewed in journals from two, usually overlapping or converging fields; and (c) those receiving a broader cross-disciplinary evaluation.

The *Mental Health Book Review Index,* 1956-1960, corresponds roughly to the review literature of 1955-1959, as selected from our group of journals. The attempt to round out our first five-year program has caused a brief delay in publishing this issue. The journals on our list have been indexed approximately to June 1960 but even then some numbers of journals current in December 1959 were not yet available. Eligible journals which only began publication in 1960 have been left for inclusion in our new program.

Beginning next year, our criteria in editing the *Index* will emphasize the multidisciplinary nature of this literature. We will then list only those books which have been reviewed in journals from three or more fields, except for books in foreign languages and those internationally reviewed, to which our former method will still be applied. While the published list of books and review citations will thus become more selective, our list of journals indexed will be kept up-to-date and our file of review references remain as comprehensive as before. Only one issue of the *Mental Health Book Review Index* will be published in 1961, in the latter half of the year; in that issue we will explain more fully our new editorial policy, which should bring us closer to a selection of significant books. Eventually, we hope to be able to show not only that the mills of the scientific community grind slowly, but also that they grind exceeding small.

# ESSAY 4

## *Book Reviewing in the Sciences of Human Behavior as a Contribution to Scholarship by the Scientific Community*

Originally published as Editorial in *Mental Health Book Review Index,* vol. 6 (whole no. 11), July 1961.

Book reviewing as a process of scholarly interaction is as old as the scientific community itself. The earliest journals, launched in the major European countries in the latter part of the 17th century, consisted primarily of book notices. They extended through print the endeavor of the academies to acquaint the learned with each other's work, and thus became one of the channels of scholarship through which the scientific community constitutes itself.

The original place of book reviews in science has been obscured, however, by later interpretations, which are still with us. One is the notion that book reviews must be either favorable or unfavorable, and when being neither, are noncommittal and somewhat amiss. This thought is borrowed from literary and art criticism and has been fostered by economic considerations. When publication is financed in advance by subsidies of learned societies, the reception of the book is primarily of scholarly interest. When books are commercially published, however, the influence of reviews upon sales becomes a matter of concern as well. It is in the spirit of science, if not always the practice, to regard book reviews as a means of extending the type of discussion that complements a paper read before a learned society. As part of the joint scientific effort, such discussion is invited to clarify and elaborate rather than to praise or disparage.

Another view of the role of book reviews in science depreciates them as a secondary source. The emphasis on facts, intensified by the positivistic movement, led to a preference for primary publications, which added new facts to the store of knowledge. When the disciplinary organization of science in the 19th century gave rise to numerous subject journals, their editors often took pride in an editorial policy that admitted only original contributions. In due course, sometimes decades later, subject journals began again to include book review sections. Nevertheless, even newly founded journals today sometimes reject book reviews on the ground that they merely summarize or discuss facts already presented.

In the sciences of human behavior, the trend which gave book reviews the status of second-class citizens in the scientific literature is being reversed. A growing number of journals in this area now have book review editors. Their editorial responsibility includes the task, first assumed in the 19th century by editors of scientific bibliographic services, of selecting significant contributions. Furthermore, rebuttals and other discussions of book reviews, traditionally tolerated, now tend to be encouraged, as in *Contemporary Psychology,* or even methodically invited, as in the *Journal of Speech and Hearing Disorders.* The tendency is not to consider the act of publishing a book complete until all three scholarly obligations, that of authors, editors, and reviewers, have been properly discharged. In this sense, the reviewers of books continue after publication the process of scientific discourse and assessment which, in the case of scientific papers and articles, involves the participation of discussants and referees before publication. The *Mental Health Book Review Index,* therefore, cites all comments and insists on including the reviewers' names in the review citations. In spite of a lingering custom of signing reviews with initials, even when the full names do not appear elsewhere in the journal, the trend away from anonymous book reviewing is unmistakable.

The behavioral sciences may be leading in this reinstatement of book reviews as a vehicle of scientific communication for a reason peculiar to them. In science, facts need to be verified, not appraised, and verification is often implicit in the very act of publication under scientific auspices. But knowledge about human nature and relations does not advance merely as an accumulation of facts and a refinement of theory. It is permeated by values, goals, and a philosophy of life. In this respect, as in others, the behavioral sciences stand between, or astride of, the natural sciences, where verification is the first requisite, and the humanities, where evaluation is the essence of critique. Therefore, when scientists and productive professional workers in the sciences of human behavior are making extensive use of journals to discuss, assess, and further each other's work published in books, they sustain, knowingly or not, a genuine tradition of the scientific community.

This idea governs everything concerning the *Mental Health Book Review Index,* its method, findings, use, and its own operational basis in the academic tradition. As a rule, where book reviews appear at all in the bibliographic record, the emphasis is on individual books. Occasionally, compilations of reviews have been designed as a guide to the literature of a limited field. Comprehensive, sustained annual bibliographies of book reviews are rare. They have not been aimed at a scholarly bibliographic synthesis. The primarily nontechnical *Book Review Digest,* published in this country since 1905, as well as the *Bibliographie der Rezensionen,* compiled in Germany from a vast number of scholarly journals, both domestic and foreign, from 1900 to 1943, have cited reviews for substantial portions of the contemporaneous book literature as a whole. Such an all-inclusive, generalized presentation does not, however, show the connection between the literature and the scholarly communities in the major areas of science, in which a meaningful exchange and interaction takes place.

In the *Mental Health Book Review Index,* we propose to restore the original conception. We believe we have demonstrated that the sciences of human behavior, which also produce the body of knowledge for the field of mental health, constitute a sector of the scientific community that is essentially stable, even though open to change. It is distinct from disciplines such as psychology, from other sectors of the scientific community such as the life sciences, and from the scientific community as a whole. The latter concept is becoming rather abstract and remote from the realities of scientific life.

The interaction, as brought into focus in the *Mental Health Book Review Index,* involves the authors who produce the body of literature, the journal editors who articulate it according to their fields of responsibility, and the reviewers, who breathe life into it by assessing the individual books in the light of their own competence and knowledge of related work. Scientific auspices, other sponsors, and commercial publishers play an essential supporting part. Neither the underlying procedures nor their implications seem to be fully understood today. The whole apparatus of book reviewing functions more on the basis of tradition and imitation than on the strength of contemporary agreements. The *Index* shows how another supporting role, not embedded in the tradition but necessary to sustain it, can be played by librarians. We believe that they, too, must contribute to a scholarly process, in whose integrity and effectiveness they are as deeply interested as the scientific community itself.

To illustrate how this may be done, we shall now present data and observations specifically derived from the *Mental Health Book Review Index*. There is, first, the evidence of the magnitude of the reviewing process in the area we survey. With the present issue, Volume 6, Whole No. 11, the *Index* completes the sixth year of its program, which now spans the period from January 1955 to May 1961. From 150 journals in the English language, which originate in eight countries in Africa, America, Australia, Asia, and Europe, we have drawn for listing in the *Index* 2,062 titles of books with a total of 10,200 references to reviews. Slightly less than one-third of the journals are published outside the United States. In this issue, they are represented in the review references in the same proportion in which they are represented in the list of journals indexed. We have found this ratio constant in all specific instances in which we have tested it, an indication of the international nature of all pertinent trends.

As noted in our list of journals indexed, book review sections and entire journals have been absorbed or discontinued, but there has been an overall trend of growth. Less than a hundred of the journals on our list have existed the whole time. Now 133 are still current, and 104 contribute an average of at least five reviews per year. The total number of books reviewed in at least one of the journals indexed is approaching 9,000. Together, these books and pamphlets on the numerous subjects relating to human behavior have elicited almost 20,000 reviews. This, in turn, is only a fraction of the books on these subjects which are concurrently being reviewed in more comprehensive scientific journals, e.g., *Science* and *Nature,* in the journals of the respective parent disciplines, and in the foreign-language and multilingual journals on the same subjects as those covered in the *Index*. Before all major criticism of significant books in the sciences of human behavior can be drawn together, we need an instrument for detecting this literature. It still remains largely submerged in the older strata of scientific organization in libraries, bibliographies, and the media of the book trade.[1] We are developing the *Mental Health Book Review Index* as such an instrument.

An underlying order suggests itself, when we look at the generations in the family of journals, as it were. Of the 20,000 review references we have gathered, 7,000 can be traced to 18 journals in, or very close to, the core subjects, psychology, psychiatry, and psychoanalysis. They fall into two groups of equal size. The first 3,500 reviews are contributed by the following six journals, here listed in the order of dates of origin: *American Journal of Psychiatry* (1844); *American Journal of Psychology* (1887/88); *Contemporary Psychology* (launched in 1956, but absorbing the reviewing function of five journals published by the American Psychological Association, the two oldest of which began in 1904 and 1906); *British Journal of Psychology* (1904/05); *International Journal of Psycho-Analysis* (1920); and *Psychoanalytic Quarterly* (1932). Their average age is 62 years. The other 3,500 reviews appeared in a group of 12 journals with an average age of 28 years, among them *Mental Hygiene* (1917); the *American Journal of Orthopsychiatry* (1930); *Psychosomatic Medicine* (1939); and the *Canadian Journal of Psychology* (1947). In contrast, 17 journals on our list, launched in 1959 or 1960, have an average age of a year and a half.

The pattern thus revealed by the *Mental Health Book Review Index* may help us to learn how to assess the machinery of assessment. The established journals which represent whole disciplines have long been supplemented by a host of journals with different orientations. The former are, however, still doing the most substantial part of the reviewing job in the behavioral sciences. They can do so because, by tradition, they command the cooperation of the specialists who must give their time and also because they receive the bulk of available review copies. The publishers cooperate partly in view of the large circulation of these journals, which, like the availability of reviewers, is guaranteed by the sponsoring or operationally related professional organizations.

Specialists working as practitioners in their respective fields will have access to one or more of the journals listed above and may consider themselves well served. Questions about the nature of this service will, however, arise among those who have scholarly responsibilities and share our concern with an encyclopedic grasp of the emerging knowledge about human behavior and its ramifications and applications in the field of mental health. To the concentration of a great many reviews in relatively few journals there corresponds a wide spread of the remainder. While 7,000 reviews can be traced to 18 journals during the period 1954/55-1960/61, the other 13,000 reviews are scattered through some 130 journals. This difference, as we have seen, is not only a numerical one. The journals which present the point of view rooted in the major disciplines as organized in the 19th and early 20th century have the most substantial book review sections and reach the largest number of readers; whereas the recent journals, which tend to be multidisciplinary from the start and often reflect a new scientific perspective, must make a greater initial effort in order to contribute to the assessment of books in the behavioral sciences and, even if they make the effort, they will not have equal opportunities to exert influence.

In addition to their advantage of easily getting the books and finding the reviewers, the older journals in psychology, psychiatry, and psychoanalysis are accessible in libraries to a degree that would be impossible to attain today. The newer journals are difficult to locate, in contrast to the established journals, which form a conspicuous part of the organized periodical literature. This constitutes an elaborate system, geared to regional, national, and international library cooperation. It comprises union lists of library holdings and library-oriented indexing services. The value of journals to libraries depends in part on their representation in periodical indexes, where the behavioral sciences, far from asserting themselves, have actually been losing ground. Until it is more fully understood how forces of inertia operate in the bibliographic organization of scientific literature, there is a danger that the use of computers, now under consideration in the library field, might further add to the unwitting reenforcement of a hierarchical structure. The *Mental Health Book Review Index* may be of help for a study of this problem.

From 1958 to 1960, the annual increment of books listed in the *Index* was fairly constant, averaging 420. This quota could only be maintained, however, by including more journals which converged in the choice of books they review with the journals in the core subjects, psychology, psychiatry, and psychoanalysis. When the latter still dominated our list of journals indexed, the number of books with one or two reviews, which we do not list, was already found to grow in geometric progression. The differential rate of growth of the titles which are listed in the *Index* and those which are not has remained constant ever since. At present, the journals on our list are evenly divided between those broadly concerned with psychology and psychotherapy, or the study of human behavior from the points of view of understanding its norms, assessing its aberrations, and healing its ills, and those concentrating on more closely defined fields of specialization within the bio-psycho-social sciences as a whole. The latter comprise journals on such subjects as child study; communication; criminology and penology, with their newer branches of criminal psychodynamics and medical and social correction; educational research; gerontology; group dynamics and human and intergroup relations; human biology, genetics, and population study; hypnosis; psychic research; rehabilitation; religious research; social problems; and social work.

When, as often happens, the old disciplinary and the new multidisciplinary journals review the same book, the approach may be totally different. The journals in psychology, psychiatry, and psychoanalysis will bring the knowledge of their disciplines to bear on assessing the book, and the range of subjects to which psychological, psychiatric, and psychoanalytic thinking and method can be applied is wide indeed. Multidisciplinary journals, on the other hand, tend to focus on one subject, topic, or even concept, e.g., alcohol and addiction, language and speech, or conflict resolution. These topical and conceptual areas of their choice they will want to illuminate with any knowledge or method that may be fruitfully applied, regardless of its disciplinary origin. In between there is another group of journals, devoted to a field of specialization, e.g., group psychotherapy. Finally, some of the journals in the new multidisciplinary areas are becoming disciplinary in their own right, as new fields, such as gerontology, reach the stage of formal scientific organization.

The cross-disciplinary reviewing as demonstrated in the *Index* must, therefore, be carefully evaluated. It does not suffice to consider a certain number of reviews of a book. For instance, books on genetics will now often be reviewed in psychological, psychiatric, and psychoanalytic journals. This does not constitute assessment of the book by the standards of science, however. The crossing of disciplinary borders sometimes implies variations in approach, at other times, degrees of competence. On a higher level, by reviewing the reviews, the scientific community must once more be the judge. Much cross-disciplinary reviewing is a way of registering interest and marks new areas of convergence. The perceptiveness shown by some editors in recognizing a new or subtle relevance to the behavioral sciences is valuable as such. It is no substitute for the discussion by a scientist speaking with authority. We submit that a "cybernetic" device such as the *Mental Health Book Review Index* may become a scholarly necessity for this reason alone. When the scientific community decides to assess the literature in concert, all the instruments must be assembled and assigned their proper place.

We have shown how the *Mental Health Book Review Index* throws light on the dimensions of book reviewing in the sciences of human behavior and on the distribution of reviews in relation to age, status, scope, and scientific orientation of the participating journals. But the magnitude of this process would be unimpressive, if it merely reflected the diffuse output of books as received from publishers. The *Index* reveals the power of direction, abstraction, discrimination, and synthesis that is generated by a superimposed intelligent effort. This is all the more notable in view of the fact that, at least so far, book reviewing in the behavioral sciences is not a concerted enterprise in the sense of planned facilitation and coordination.

A few examples may illustrate this point. This issue contains about 300 titles of books listed in the *Index* for the first time, and about 100 listed in previous issues, for which groups of three or more reviews are now cited for the second, third, or fourth time. Among these 400 titles, two areas of concentration stand out. One refers to subject matter. Approximately every fifth book is concerned with children or adolescents. This is out of proportion to the small number of journals on our list specifically devoted to child psychology and psychiatry. This subject emphasis in the assessment of the monographic literature may reflect a striving of the scientific community to overcome the effects of divided knowledge and competence according to professional affiliation in a field where such artificial separation proves to be particularly damaging. The *Mental Health Book Review Index* may here serve as a pilot bibliography and assist those planning to advance and consolidate the scientific organization directed to the study of the child, through new training programs, scientific societies, encyclopedic works, and journals open to contributions from all pertinent disciplines and professions.

The other area of concentration refers to a type of publication that may be categorized as "stock-taking." Scientific progress has two major phases. After an advance into new territory, a reviewing sets in which aims at a comprehensive and systematic presentation of the results. What used to be new knowledge then becomes background knowledge. To a degree, this is a continuous process. The present issue of the *Index* suggests, however, that here, too, major trends may come into play which we have as yet failed to master with the scientific method.

Roughly every fourth book listed in this issue of the *Index* might be claimed by this category of stock-taking. It comprises such types of publications as histories; books on the theory and fundamentals of a field; inventories of research, reviews and bibliographies; monographs concerned with training and methodology; selected papers, classics, and books presenting the fruits of a scientist's life work. Conspicuous works in this category are the major handbooks with an encyclopedic scope or intent which require so much preparation and support that they cannot be produced too often within a scientific generation.

A year ago we listed in Issue no. 10 of the *Index* handbooks in the fields of neurophysiology,[2] psychology,[3] and clinical psychology.[4] The present issue adds to those a handbook on psychiatry,[5] two on aging produced under the auspices of the Inter-University Council, later the Inter-University Training Institute in Social Gerontology,[6,7] the third volume of Study 1 of *Psychology: a Study of a Science,* sponsored by the American Psychological Association with support from the National Science Foundation,[8] and, on a more limited scale, handbooks on epilepsy,[9] pharmacopsychology,[10] and neurological diagnostic methods.[11]

This seems like a harvest for which the seeds must have been planted years and even decades ago. The evidence presented by the *Mental Health Book Review Index* that so many initially unrelated undertakings are now before the scientific community for assessment is timely. The mental health movement, in its eagerness to promote research as well as in its concern with mental health education, has reached a stage of self-criticism, which tends to take the form of a quest for "bodies of knowledge." Even the term "mental health" has been challenged on the ground that it does not represent a body of knowledge, as did "mental hygiene." While the awareness of an increasingly intolerable lack in the access to knowledge is sound, there seems to be no clear understanding of its nature. "Mental health" can be as useful a term as "mental hygiene" to designate a body of knowledge, provided an effort is made to identify, organize, and present the literature comprising this body of knowledge.

We began six years ago to make such an effort. As a result, the term "mental health" can now be used to refer not only to a body of knowledge in the traditional sense, but to a body of knowledge which, like man himself, is subject to an evolutionary process and developing its potential for self-awareness and self-direction. What has been found wanting is neither the production of literature, whether of the exploratory or the stock-taking type, nor the provisions for its assessment, but rather an understanding of their nature and of the need for fundamental adjustments which would narrow, although they can never close, the gap between organization and advancement of the sciences of human behavior.

A major gap exists not in the body of knowledge and the primary channels for communicating it, but in the methods and procedures used by libraries and literature services. They operate within a framework of scientific organization which allows them to absorb the literature of the behavioral sciences, but not to present it in a scientifically meaningful way. We have tried, in the *Index,* to document our analysis of the problem and to trace it to its roots. We have also experimented with a new principle of organizing this literature. It develops the idea that the sciences most intimately concerned with the study of human behavior, which we call the core subjects, psychology, psychiatry, and psychoanalysis, must be placed in the center of the new structure for the literature relating to human behavior. Contributions from allied and converging fields will fall in order in various positions governed by laws not yet brought under the command of scientific understanding.

Our present editorial policy carries this experiment a step farther. In the preceding ten issues of the *Index,* January 1956 to July 1960, we listed books with any three or more references to reviews. In this issue, this procedure has been retained in the following instances: when the three or more reviews appear in any of the psychological, psychiatric, or psychoanalytic journals indexed; when the reviews appear in at least three journals originating outside the United States; or when the books reviewed are in foreign languages. However, if none of these criteria are met, books are listed only when the journals contributing reviews represent at least three different fields, which may entail a combination of journals in the core subjects with those in the peripheral fields or combinations of the latter among themselves. At this time, fifty titles of books with three or more reviews failed to meet any of these criteria; two thirds of their reviews appear in journals in the fields of criminology and social work.

Through this procedure we hope to be able to study more closely the emergence of the sciences of human behavior as a new development in science. It is often said that science is international, but this statement needs clarification. Fundamentally, science is cosmopolitan, directed to a universal search for truth without boundaries of any kind. The organization of science, however, recognizes many boundaries. In the 19th century, there was a tendency to organize science simultaneously within disciplinary and national borders and then to provide for international cooperation among scientists in the same disciplines. This vulnerable structure still prevails in the behavioral sciences, which have their origin in the 19th century and were influenced by its ideology. The multidisciplinary development, which is now being superimposed upon the disciplinary structure, is at the same time supranational in its orientation. Our editorial policy aims at a clearer understanding of the literature of the behavioral sciences as a whole by emphasizing the three-fold disciplinary background as well as the problems involved in trying to transcend borders, both of countries and of disciplines.

So far we have talked only about the books and review references listed in the *Index*, but have not even mentioned the reviews themselves. It goes without saying that they constitute a resource of extraordinary potential. We have laid it open for use. The contribution we offer as librarians consists primarily in bringing the scattered and elusive reviews back to the state of ready reference and high visibility which any assessment must have. The bibliography of book reviews, based on an indirect method of selection, would now have to be turned over to the scholars in the sciences of human behavior for an assessment of the reviews and a definitive selection. In essence, this would merely repeat on a higher level, and in a sense restore, the cumulative process basic to science.

For a start, it would seem to be particularly profitable to study and summarize the reviews directed to the 25 percent or so of the books which have or make a claim to being used as standard and reference works. A study of the reviews of conference proceedings and research, also amply presented in the *Index*, may become a useful guide for the sponsoring organizations. In general, the academic community and the grant-giving foundations and government agencies, which are concerned about the most effective use of available funds, might be interested in seeing how work that was so amply promoted during the past decade now stands up under the scrutiny of the scientific community.

Many more questions might be raised, which could be answered by our data under appropriate conditions of research. For example, there is a striking difference between the ease and speed with which books in the area of social psychiatry and medical sociology can be put in evidence in the *Index*, and the failure of a good many books in the field of social psychology to meet the same criteria for listing. The *Index* shows how methodically psychological journals contribute in general to the assessment of books pertaining to their various specialties, but *Contemporary Psychology* appears to be virtually alone in assuming responsibility for reviewing books on social psychology. Specialists working in such fields as race problems and minority relations appear to be unaware of the fact that this difference exists and of the further discrepancies to which it may lead. What they hope to achieve in the realm of research and social action may remain unrecognized in the realm of library and literature services, where their work is not adequately represented. Such lacunae in the scholarly record should be examined. They can often be traced to policies and procedures which may need to be reconsidered and revised.

Our proposal to bring the power of consensus, controversy, and cross-disciplinary comment and criticism to bear on the problem of structuring the literature of the behavioral sciences and the field of mental health is now in itself before the scientific community for assessment. The bibliographic demonstration, showing that the literature of the sciences of human behavior is indeed a distinctive one, cutting across the biological, psychological, and sociological disciplines as well as the professional fields which further criss-cross the same area, is corroborated by a negative test. There has been a trend, which began about ten years ago, to take the literature of the behavioral sciences out of more comprehensive literature services in which they used to hold a place. Where programs start or change with a view to solving current problems of scientific information, the behavioral sciences tend to be left out. This sector of the scientific community is evidently expected to take care of its own more delicate problems of organizing its literature. But this has not been the case. The assumption that it can be and is being done through disciplinary channels lingers on, although it is obviously no longer valid. At present, the *Mental Health Book Review Index* represents the only effort to approach the problem from the vantage point of the behavioral sciences and the field of mental health as a whole, and to anchor this approach at the same time in the scholarly channels of the library field and the scientific community.

This issue of the *Mental Health Book Review Index* has again been compiled and edited by librarians working without special funds, but with the resources available to those who stay within the scholarly channels of librarianship and science. We submit it in the belief that it may enhance the contribution to scholarship, made by the scientific community through the assessment of books in the sciences of human behavior. In addition, we hope that the *Mental Health Book Review Index,* and this issue in particular, may help to clear the ground for a development which we regard as necessary and even urgent indeed. This is the recognition of the study of the literature in the sciences of human behavior as a legitimate field for research, teaching, scientific theory, and useful application.

## REFERENCES AND NOTES

1. Editorial: The behavioral sciences and mental health in relation to the organization of knowledge, the organization of science, and bibliography. See this volume, p. 9.

2. *Handbook of physiology; a critical comprehensive presentation of physiological knowledge and concepts.* Section 1: Neurophysiology. John Field, editor-in-chief, H. W. Magoun, section editor, Victor E. Hall, executive editor. Washington, American Physiological Society. Distributors: Baltimore, Williams & Wilkins; London, Baillière, Tindall & Cox, 1959-1960. 2 v.

3. *Psychology: a study of a science.* Study 1: Conceptual and systematic. Vol. 1: Sensory, perceptual, and physiological formations. Ed. by Sigmund Koch. N.Y., London, McGraw-Hill, 1959. 710 pp.

4. Stern, Erich, ed. *Handbuch der klinischen Psychologie.* Bd. 2: Die Psychotherapie in der Gegenwart; Richtungen, Aufgaben, Probleme, Anwendungen. Hrsg. unter Mitarbeit von E. Blum et al. Zürich, Rascher, 1958. 474 pp.

5. *American handbook of psychiatry.* Silvano Arieti, editor. Editorial board: Kenneth E. Appel, Daniel Blain, Norman Cameron, Kurt Goldstein, and Lawrence C. Kolb. N.Y., Basic Books; London, Mayflower, 1959. 2 v (2098 pp.)

6. *Handbook of aging and the individual; psychological and biological aspects.* Ed. by James E. Birren. Editorial committee: John E. Anderson, Ewald W. Busse, and Albert I. Lansing. Under the auspices of the Inter-University Council on Social Gerontology. [Companion volume to *Handbook of social gerontology,* ed. by Clark Tibbits.] Chicago, Univ. of Chicago Pr.; London, Cambridge Univ. Pr., 1960. 939 pp.

7. Tibbits, Clark, ed. *Handbook of social gerontology; societal aspects of aging.* Editorial board: Ernest W. Burgess, John W. McConnell, and Leo W. Simmons. Foreword by Wilma Donahue. Under the auspices of the Inter-University Training Institute in Social Gerontology. [Companion volume to *Handbook of aging and the individual,* ed. by James E. Birren.] Chicago, Univ. of Chicago Pr.; London, Cambridge Univ. Pr., 1960. 770 pp.

8. *Psychology: a study of a science.* Study 1: Conceptual and systematic. Vol. 3: Formulations of the person and the social context. Ed. by Sigmund Koch. N.Y., London, McGraw-Hill, 1959. 837 pp.

9. Lennox, William Gordon. *Epilepsy and related disorders.* With the collaboration of Margaret A. Lennox. Boston, Little, Brown; London, Churchill, 1960. 2 v. (1168 pp.)

10. Lippert, Herbert. *Einführung in die Pharmakopsychologie.* Bern, Stuttgart, Huber, 1959. 254 pp. (Enzyklopädie der Psychologie in Einzeldarstellungen, Bd. 4).

11. McDowell, Fletcher, and Wolff, Harold G., eds. *Handbook of neurological diagnostic methods.* [Based on the collaboration of the members of the Neurological Division of the Department of Medicine of Cornell University Medical College.] Baltimore, Williams & Wilkins; London, Baillière, Tindall & Cox, 1960. 201 pp.

# ESSAY 5

## *The Conservation of Knowledge about Human Behavior*

Originally published as Editorial in *Mental Health Book Review Index,* vol. 7 (whole no. 12), 1962.

One of the changes brought about by the atomic and space age is the organized linking of science with public policy and action. Fallout and space probes were soon recognized as matters of joint concern to scientists, government, and the public. More slowly, mental health, the behavioral sciences, and scientific information have also become public issues. Each of these is now seen as a separate critical area. But we recognize their problems as interrelated and get a bird's-eye view of the situation as a whole, when we turn to another matter of common interest. This is the conservation of knowledge evolving from the behavioral sciences in interaction with the field of mental health.

To conserve knowledge and thereby to sustain intellectual and cultural continuity has always been the scholar's concern, whether he be scientist, teacher, editor, or librarian. Many scientists wish to pursue and to share knowledge, but give little thought to the ways by which it might be conserved. The documentation movement seeks to adapt the processes of conservation to modern technology and has focused on the storage and retrieval of information. As mechanization proceeds, the units become smaller, their speed is accelerated, and the particles eligible for storage, although almost too perishable for that, multiply at an exponential rate.

In the *Mental Health Book Review Index* we have been guided by the scholarly goal, which bids those who will pursue it to make haste slowly. We have asked: when do organic parts of knowledge form larger units; where, in the behavioral sciences and the field of mental health, are such larger units further synthesized; and how can we get hold of a body of knowledge that is to be conserved and integrated with the main current of human endeavor in our time?

Leaving technological problems to those already engaged in efforts to solve them, we have considered other steps that may follow from changes in the concept of scientific truth. In modern science, knowledge is never regarded as final; it is constantly being revised, refined, possibly reversed, and it cannot be halted or frozen at any point. Methods designed to conserve knowledge about human behavior must, therefore, be fluid and dynamic. It does not follow that we must retain all particles for continuous rearrangements. We may strive for a synthesis, provided we do not present it as final.

The *Mental Health Book Review Index* uses journals as its starting point, as do most indexing and abstracting services. But here we part company. The scientific information services analyze the body of the journals, but omit book reviews, unless these appear as articles. We do the opposite. We include articles only when they deal with books, index all book review sections, and make an effort to note any other comments on monographic publications made anywhere in a journal by editors, authors, or readers.

The list of journals we index has been kept open to include additional and newly launched periodicals related to the behavioral sciences and the field of mental health. More than one third of the 170 journals in the English language that we have indexed since 1954/55 began publication during this period. Now 145 of them are still current and continue to serve as media for book reviews. During the past seven years, these journals have published almost 24,000 reviews of about 10,500 books and pamphlets. However, the reviews have not been evenly distributed at any time. About half of them tend to form clusters around only one fourth of all the books reviewed; for the other books the critical discussion is spread rather thin.

For further study we have concentrated on the titles reviewed in at least three of the journals indexed, holding the others in abeyance in our files. Twice a year from 1956 to 1960 and annually since, we have listed books with references to three or more reviews. They are mostly drawn from journals representing the psychological sciences, psychology, psychiatry, and psychoanalysis, which we regard as the core subjects of the behavioral sciences. For the listing of books primarily reviewed in journals from allied fields, we have tightened and refined our criteria. We are concerned with the literature contributing to the common goal, the understanding of human behavior. In the present Volume 7 of the *Index,* we list books reviewed in journals from various other fields only when we can also cite at least one review from a journal in any of the psychological sciences.

An annual volume of the *Index* now covers about 400 books currently under review in the fields which our journals represent. About 80 percent of these titles appear in the *Index* for the first time. For the books previously listed we add groups of three or more review citations. Some books are thus listed for several years, over and over again. Many of these may turn out to be landmarks in the pursuit of knowledge.

The fact that the number of books listed in the *Index* increases arithmetically, not in the dreaded geometric progression, may be felt as a relief, but this in itself would not bring us closer to our aim. The question remains whether the almost 2,400 books listed in the *Index* with 12,000 references to reviews differ in quality from the more than 8,000 books which attracted only limited or scattered attention in the same group of journals. A full evaluation of individual books may result from the "reviewing of reviews," which we recommend. We can, however, note certain characteristics by simply looking at our bibliographic data.

The books listed include those that are most substantial. We find here the pertinent publications of recent years which have themselves reviewed, reported, and condensed large amounts of knowledge: the comprehensive handbooks and other reference works, textbooks and methodological guides, literature studies, conference proceedings, and major surveys conducted with government or foundation support. A key to the emerging editorial and critical opinion expressed in representative subject journals, as offered by the *Index,* may be especially useful when such documents are before Congress and the public, as is now the case with the Final Report of the Joint Commission on Mental Illness and Health, entitled *Action for Mental Health.*

The mass of data behind a publication is not the only yardstick to its significance. The reviewing process may also be described as a scouting for novel ideas and subtle connections. A new current of thought such as existentialism or the scientific study of religion may prompt specialists to reinterpret a book not previously reviewed in this light. A cultural trend in favor of integrative approaches may affect ways of dealing with emotional and political tensions and at the same time direct the reviewers' interest to books on family and community relations, conflict resolution, and character development. Social concern can also express itself, for instance, through the growing number of reviews of paperback editions, aimed at students and the general public. Certain broad topics such as the study of children and adolescents, education, delinquency and mental subnormality, human genetics, psychopharmacology, social psychiatry, communication, group relations, social welfare, rehabilitation, and aging, keep recurring, but it is possible to trace changes in emphasis through the clustering of book reviews, which pick out specific titles.

How is this selection achieved? Basically, by an invisible panel of judges who never met for this purpose and, for all we know, are unaware of each other's participation. We are reminded of the "Invisible College," which more than three hundred years ago helped to bring the modern scientific community into being.

The judges, to a considerable extent, represent the scientific community in the behavioral sciences. Many of the reviewers have editorial responsibilities for leading journals in the various fields, including the function of book review editor, mentioned in an earlier editorial as a noteworthy development in the literature of science. Many books are reviewed by authorities on the subject. It would appear that the more significant the books, the better the chances that they will be reviewed by the author's elders and peers. By the same token, the reviewers' rank in the scientific community suggests the rank of the work under review, although the marshalling of notable names need not signify a salute. In addition to its current value, the critical discussion of an important work contributes to the history of ideas.

In a previous editorial[1] we gave some reasons why there is no place for the sciences of human behavior and the field of mental health in the present structure of organized science. The critical evaluation of books by the scientific community helps to overcome this difficulty. The concerted effort may be viewed as a system without a tangible structure, which serves the functional needs of the psychological and behavioral sciences and allied professions. No one directs, instructs, or coordinates this system. Its self-organizing principle is the intrinsic goal, to unify knowledge about man.

It is not incidental but vital for such a system, so long as its needs run counter to the machinery of managerial support, that it can depend upon the tradition of scholarly exchange. In this whole book reviewing process no money changes hands; the benefits take another form. Publishers provide the review copies, on their own initiative or upon request. Their cooperation is rewarded by a review, or acknowledged in a list of books received. It is the reviewer's compensation that he may keep the book. Thus the intellectual process of distilling knowledge consumes, but does not conserve the books and monographs as physical literature. To complete the conservation of knowledge initiated by publishers and furthered by editors and reviewers, it is necessary to call upon librarians, who will contribute the bibliographic synthesis and make the significant literature available.

At present the contribution of organized librarianship toward that end is almost as invisible as the contribution of the scientific community. No single library is designated to serve the behavioral sciences and the field of mental health; none has even all the journals we index or all the books we list. We can find them, however, in the library system as a whole. In this country, the printed National Union Catalog, which incorporates the catalog cards of the Library of Congress and the National Library of Medicine, unifies the bibliographic information further contributed by the cooperating academic, research, and public libraries in the United States and Canada. When the *Mental Health Book Review Index* lists the books identified as pertinent and selected for evaluation by the scientific community throughout the English-speaking world, the basic cataloging work for these books has already been done in a form accepted by libraries in this country and many others overseas. The editors of the *Index* often give more detailed cataloging information. Nevertheless, the organized library system provides the bibliographic nucleus, just as the scientific community provides the basis for our selection.

The *Mental Health Book Review Index,* like everything else connected with this reviewing process, is sustained by scholarly exchanges. Operating without financial support, it derives its main capacity to function from the harnessing of human brain power. The intellectual energy which flows into the book reviews and the library catalogs is not exhausted in these channels. The *Index* uses the extraordinary potential of this intellectual power for the purpose of creating an integrated bibliography. Neither the scientific community nor the library system, each limited to its own resources, would be in a position to produce such a bibliography. But both have contributed most of the necessary human power, and both may benefit from the *Index*.

## NOTES

1. The Behavioral Sciences and Mental Health in Relation to the Organization of Knowledge, the Organization of Science, and Bibliography. See this volume, p. 9.

# ESSAY 6

## *Changes in the Concept of "Scientific Literature"*

Originally published as Editorial in *Mental Health Book Review Index,* vol. 8 (whole no. 13), 1963. Reprinted in *College and Research Libraries,* vol. 25, no. 4, January 1964, pp. 27-31. Reprinted here with References and Notes from *Journal of the History of the Behavioral Sciences,* vol. 1, no. 3, July 1965, pp. 235-243.

The current concern with the fate of scientific writings is not new, but new is the shift of emphasis which has put *information,* not *literature,* in the center of attention. We may wonder what has happened to the literature of science. Has it been superseded by the computer? Or have we, in the excitement over acquiring a gigantic robot memory, suffered a lapse of our human memory and lost sight of scientific literature as a cultural possession?

### DIVORCE OF SCIENCE FROM LITERATURE

At the dawn of Western civilization, literature and science were intimately linked. Literature not only absorbed the thought of its time, but could express insights that foreshadowed a knowledge yet to come. Thus Lucretius' poem, *De Rerum Natura,* has been acclaimed for showing an amazing foreknowledge of atomic science and electronics.[1] This unity of literature and science lasted as long as a unifying view of the world prevailed. The kinship between the ideas of poets and the poetic response of men of science, still strong in contemporaries like Donne and Kepler, then gave way to a new spirit, which severed modern science from literature as an art.[2]

De Quincey was the first to delimit literature clearly as a fine art, excluding from it "all books in which the matter to be communicated is paramount to the manner or form of its communication" and, therefore, excluding "all *science* whatsoever." Thus the expulsion of science from literature became an explicit part of literary theory. De Quincey was aware, however, that the common use of the word *literature* was not as discriminating as he would have it: "Popularly, and amongst the thoughtless, it is held to include everything that is printed in a book," or it was "a mere term of convenience for expressing inclusively the total books in a language." In a philosophical sense, he asserted, it would be ludicrous to reckon a pharmacopoeia, the Court Calendar, etc., as part of the literature.[3]

Throughout the remainder of the 19th century, dictionaries, in their definitions of literature, reflected the adoption of De Quincey's perceptive distinctions, but without retaining his value judgments. In the 1860's it became necessary to record another meaning: "the whole body of literary productions or writings upon a given subject, or in reference to a particular science or branch of knowledge."[4] Thus, in relation to scientific writings in a given field, literature was now again defined in the single, all-inclusive sense which De Quincey had branded as popular, thoughtless, and ludicrous.

## FREEZING AN OBSOLETE STRUCTURE

At the turn of the century science paid a heavy price for being cut off from the humanities and social sciences, with their longer vistas and openness to social and intellectual history. The 19th-century structure of disciplines, each thought of as having a literature of its own, was frozen into 20th-century scientific bibliography. This meant that a concept of "scientific literature" which was static, rigid, and aloof, gained acceptance at the very time when science itself became more than ever dynamic, fluid, and exposed to interaction with the social scene.

There had been no such conflict so long as the concern with scientific writings was retrospective, as, for example, in the Royal Society's *Catalogue of Scientific Papers, 1800-1900,* and in a corresponding French national bibliography.[5] In that case plans drawn up at mid-century were still useful, when the work came to fruition at the *fin de siècle.* Different problems arose, however, when the *International Catalogue of Scientific Literature* was launched as an enormous project of international cooperation. It called for "a complete index of current scientific literature," beginning with the year 1901. The basic subject arrangement corresponded to the then recognized disciplines in the exact sciences. It was also felt "that an authors' catalogue could not supply the required information, and that it was essential that scientific workers should be kept fully and quickly informed of all new discoveries by means of complete subject indexes."[6] Neither the implicit assumption nor the language appear to have changed very much over the past sixty years in the planning of comprehensive, current scientific information services.

It was also around 1900 that a new era began for certain fields of science, for instance, the atomic sciences, genetics, and psychoanalysis. The *International Catalogue of Scientific Literature* achieved on a worldwide scale what would now be called the coordination of scientific information. Here we have the ingredients of a scholarly study laid out for us. We might ask, for example, how new discoveries, as now recognized, found their way to other scientific workers; what else besides information was involved in their further development and acceptance; what this monumental index of current scientific literature actually contributed to the advancement of scientific knowledge, and at what price. By raising this last question, we do not mean the cost in terms of money and manpower, although this, too, may be of interest today. Rather, we refer to the retarding and inhibiting influences which can now be traced to the *International Catalogue.* The undertaking, which commanded the authority and resources of its time, has left its mark on bibliographic and library organization up to the present day.[7]

The *Bibliographie der deutschen naturwissenschaftlichen Litteratur,* also launched in 1901 to report in brief intervals the German material contributed to the annually published *International Catalogue,* but otherwise coordinated with it, permits a close view of the intellectual strait jacket sanctioned by international consent. The ingenuity with which works in the then emerging behavioral sciences were pressed into a scheme already obsolete at its inception is especially remarkable, but it is also deceptive. We might not think of looking in a bibliography severely limited to the exact sciences for the third German edition of Eugen Dühring's *The Marquis de Sade and His Time; Studies in the History of Culture and Morals of the Eighteenth Century.* Yet there it is, listed under "Physiology of Reproduction," with a cross reference from "Nervous System."[8] Such examples might be multiplied, but it is more important to stress the principle: an index of the world's current scientific literature can be *current* only if it is organized within the framework of the contemporaneous trends in scientific thinking and research.

An international convention with the power to reconsider and, if necessary, to revise the regulations and schedules approved for the *International Catalogue,* was to be held in 1905, in 1910, and every tenth year afterwards. This liberal foresight was of no avail; publication, interrupted in 1915-16, ceased in 1921 with Volume 254. Even then disillusionment appears to have tempered regret. In a comprehensive address on "The Record of Science," published in *Science,* a leading American librarian, William Warner Bishop, noted briefly that this great international undertaking that was to be the final word in all branches of pure science was already breaking down of its own weight before the World War, which then brought it to a halt. Of the "huge series of annual volumes" Bishop had only this to say: "The set remains a monument to the difficulties of the task of an adequate index to the published work of scientists."[9] Four decades later its greatest value might be in helping us to recognize it as 'a monument to the dangers' of attempting to freeze science and, in particular, to the paradox of building obsolete concepts of scientific literature into a new bibliographic system under the guise of the latest advances in information systems management and engineering.

## A NEW LITERARY THEORY FOR SCIENCE

During the past fifty years the link between science and literature that was broken by the rise of modern science in the 17th century has begun to be restored. First, there have been significant changes in literary theory. Among the leading ideas here are that literature and science are inseparable expressions of the creative human spirit and that, while the working processes of science are indeed incompatible with literature, mankind becomes conscious of itself through literature which is both science and art. It has also been fully recognized that science has had an all-pervading influence upon modern literature, which in turn becomes the vehicle through which science affects men's whole lives and their modes of thought, emotion, and action; and that science has directly contributed works of the highest rank to literature.[10]

A history of scientific literature, based on criteria of value, was first clearly envisaged in 1930 in the dissertation, *Studies in the Literature of Natural Science,* by J. M. Drachman. The idea of such a history has since gained in breadth and depth. The progress made may, however, be concealed behind a disclaimer, as in Grant McColley's *Literature and Science; an Anthology from English and American Literature, 1600-1900,* or behind titles which still avoid the word *literature* in the context of *science,* such as *Books That Changed Our Minds, Books That Changed the World,* or *Molders of the Moden Mind; 111 Books That Shaped Western Civilization.*[11]

Furthermore, we may consider the diversity of forms of writing and publication as a matrix for scientific literature. The past fifty or a hundred years were rich in developments which, while provoking some reaction in the humanities, have gone almost unnoticed in science, for instance, the Festschrift, the invited lecture, the prize essay, the editorial and letter to the editor, the book review and rebuttal, the selected bibliography, and the monographic series or single book appearing under the editorship of a distinguished scholar or scientist.[12] Not only has little been done to study their place and function in scientific discourse, but they are usually omitted from the major scientific information services, which tend to limit themselves to journals and proceedings, technical reports, and sometimes monographs, the material that lends itself to routine processes. Yet those more elusive forms of scholarly presentation have become sensitive instruments, when put at the disposal of the scientific community. Its members often choose these channels to transmit their germinal ideas, their scientific philosophy and theoretical probings, their standards, judgments, and concerns, their wisdom as elder statesmen, in short, the currents of scientific thought and scholarship which give meaning and direction to the minutiae of research and compensate for the narrowing confines imposed by specialization.

## THE RISE OF SCIENTIFIC JOURNALISM

In order to develop a concept of scientific literature for our time, we may have to reinterpret a type of publication which serves only the purpose of providing scientific information. This "scientific journalism" spreads as much scientific knowledge as can be reasonably absorbed and digested through the self-organizing audiences reached by the individual journals; it therefore calls into service a large number of scientists with varying editorial responsibilities, who see to it that the dissemination of knowledge remains authentic and stimulating, qualities sometimes diluted or lost in abstracting and indexing. With the spread of scientific literacy, the number of authors and readers of scientific writings has been vastly enlarged. Scientific journalism affords an outlet for communications on scientific subjects, which are not necessarily contributions to scientific knowledge.[13] At the same time, this form of publication generates a continued discussion, often followed by republication, of outstanding contributions, which will eventually find their way into scientific literature. As a reservoir of scientific information that can be of significance to the nonspecialist and the lay public, scientific journalism is also linked with journalism in general through the work of professional science writers.

## THE CRITIC AS LIBERATOR

In a positive way, the literature of science can crystallize only after a scholarly criticism of scientific writings has fully emerged.[14] One task of such criticism is to clarify what each form of scientific presentation can contribute to the body of literature as a whole; another, to analyze the intrinsic rules imposed upon the literature by the nature of scientific inquiry in various areas of science. Most important is the scientist's responsibility, in his capacity as critic, to recognize and select from the flow of publications those works that meet the highest standards.

A beginning toward organized criticism in science was made in the annual reviews and review articles. Now scientific book reviews, often discredited in the older disciplines, appear to be gaining.[15] In multidisciplinary areas, in particular, book reviews which throw light upon a work from the various interlocking fields can point the way from an indiscriminate mass of scientific writings to scientific literature. When critical judgments are pooled and receive bibliographic recognition over a sustained period, it becomes apparent that such collective criticism tends to sift and to lift out the works that are substantial, articulate, and mature.[16] This process can shorten the time needed for a selection of contemporary scientific literature. Just as, in the words of Joseph de Maistre, "Chaque nation est pour l'autre une postérité contemporaine,"[17] so can each related discipline be a discerning critic for another. Once established, criticism in science should find its own form of expression. It can then make scientific literature, as R. A. Scott-James put it for the relation of literary criticism to literature in general, "self-conscious about itself, about its own processes, its technique, its aim."[18]

## CONCEPTUAL ROOTS OF THE CRISIS

In a critique of current scientific periodical articles as a literature lacking in literary values, John Maddox has raised the crucial question: "Is the Literature Worth Keeping?"[19] We believe that what deserves to be called literature in science is worth keeping, but it is not limited to any single form of writing or confined to a channel that has become obvious, outworn, and wide-open. Nor need we look for this literature in the machines that may eventually assist us in recording it.

A chiefly technological approach has been promoted for about twenty years now, and yet the "crisis in scientific information" has been aggravated rather than relieved.[20] Underlying this crisis is the lingering use of a concept of scientific literature which was new in the latter part of the 19th century. It was a misunderstanding to apply this concept directly to the bibliography of 20th-century science by merely trying to list *all current publications in a given field.*

The time has come to cultivate a concern over the *evolving contemporary scientific literature,* and to develop adequate bibliographic methods through a scholarly approach. This need not be done in an atmosphere of crisis. By taking the longer view of the historian, the humanist, and the librarian, we can see even now that some problems of scientific information storage and retrieval seem to defy solution because they do not need one. For information that does not contribute to scientific knowledge is not worth retrieving, and the only indestructible way of storing scientific knowledge is by allowing it to become scientific literature, and by helping it to become so recognized and known.

## REFERENCES AND NOTES

1. M. D. C. Tait, "Lucretius," *University of Toronto Quarterly* 2, 21 (1932); C. Bailey, "Lucretius," annual lecture on a master mind, Henriette Hertz Trust, *Proc. Brit. Acad. London* 35, 143 (1949); also published separately, (Cumberlege, London, 1949); M. Moore, "Concerning the creative process in literature," in *Experimental Psychopathology,* P. H. Hoch and J. Zubin, Eds., (Grune & Stratton, New York, 1957), p. 122; G. Müller, *Die Darstellung der Kinetik bei Lukrez* (Akademie-Verlag, Berlin, 1959), p. 117; A. Gerlo, *Lukrez, Gipfel der antiken Atomistik* (Akademie-Verlag, Berlin, 1961), pp. 7, 13-14; A. D. Winspear, *Lucretius and Scientific Thought* (Harvest House, Montreal, 1963), pp. 80-117.

2. C. S. Duncan, *The New Science and English Literature in the Classical Period,* thesis, Univ. of Chicago (Banta Publishing Co., Menasha, Wisconsin, 1913); D. Bush, *Science and English Poetry: a Historical Sketch, 1590-1950* (Oxford Univ. Press, New York, 1950), pp. 27-50; R. F. Jones, "Science and criticism in the neo-classical age of English literature"; "Science and English prose style in the third quarter of the seventeenth century," in *The Seventeenth Century: Studies in the History of English Thought and Literature from Bacon to Pope by Richard Foster Jones and Others Writing in His Honor* (Stanford Univ. Press, Stanford, 1961), pp. 41-74, 75-110; M. H. Nicolson, *The Breaking of the Circle: Studies in the Effect of the "New Science" upon Seventeenth-Century Poetry* (Columbia Univ. Press, New York, rev. ed., 1960), pp. 123-165; D. Bush, "Science and literature," in *Seventeenth Century Science and the Arts,* the William J. Cooper Foundation lectures, Swarthmore College, 1960, H. H. Rhys, Ed., (Princeton Univ. Press, Princeton, 1961), pp. 29-62.

3. T. De Quincey, "Letters to a young man whose education has been neglected" (1823), in *The Collected Writings of Thomas De Quincey,* D. Masson, Ed., (Black, Edinburgh, new and enlarged ed., 1890), vol. 10, pp. 14, 17; ——, "The poetry of Pope" (1848), *ibid.,* vol. 11, p. 53; S. K. Proctor, *Thomas De Quincey's Theory of Literature* (Univ. of Michigan Press, Ann Arbor, 1943), pp. 107-122.

4. The 18th-century definition of literature given by Johnson as "learning; skill in letters" was retained as the only one into the 19th century, when it meant a knowledge of the humanities "as well as of the sciences" (Webster, 1828). The next definition added to it was "the collective body of literary productions, embracing the entire results of knowledge and fancy preserved in writing." Under the influence of De Quincey's literary theory both definitions were narrowed to exclude

explicitly the positive or physical sciences (Webster, 1840); Worcester, 1846). Distinction in thought, style, and artistic construction gradually became a criterion in defining literature other than science. The "thoroughly revised" 1864 edition of Webster's *American Dictionary of the English Language* appears to have been the first to introduce the new definition relating literature specifically to a given subject or a particular science or branch of knowledge. In 1905, the *Oxford English Dictionary,* limiting this usage to "the body of books and writings that treat of a particular subject," gives 1860 and 1879 as the earliest dates to which it can be traced. A clear statement of the consensus that had been reached before 1900 appears in C. F. Johnson, *Elements of Literary Criticism* (Harper, New York and London, 1898), p. 1: ". . . the word Literature is very much changed in extent and significance by its qualifying adjective. Thus, if we should say, 'The Literature of Chemistry,' or 'The Literature of Geology,' we should mean all that has been written on these sciences . . . If, however, we should use the term 'English Literature,' we should by no means wish to include all that has been written or printed in the English language." See also (*12*).

5. J. Deniker, *Bibliographies des travaux scientifiques (sciences mathématiques, physiques et naturelles) publiés par les sociétés savantes de la France depuis l'origine jusqu'en 1888,* dressés sous les auspices du Ministère de l'instruction publique (Imprimerie Nationale, Paris, 1895-1922), 2 vols.

6. *International Catalogue of Scientific Literature* . . . 1901-1914 (Published for the International Council by the Royal Society of London, London, 1902-1921), 254 vols., preface to each volume of the first annual issue, p. v. In view of recurrent attempts to offer similar ideas as innovations, the details of this historic proposal deserve to be recalled: "In order that a scientific investigator might be in a position to ascertain by means of the Catalogue what has from time to time been published concerning each particular subject of inquiry, it was held to be of great importance that not only the titles of papers but their subject matter also should be indexed. As stated above, however, financial considerations have led to the number of subject-entries being at present limited in number. But the expense of making subject-entries would be very greatly reduced if all periodicals adopted a practice already carried out by some journals, namely, that of indexing each paper at the time of its publication. Indeed, were this carefully done, the Bureaus preparing the Catalogue would no longer have to study the contents of papers in order to prepare the subject-entries, and the saving thereby effected would make it possible to enlarge the scope of the Catalogue, until it include all original scientific communications. Seeing how necessary such a

complete subject catalogue is for the progress of science, it is hoped that all editors and authors will co-operate in so preparing subject-indexes for all papers at the time of their publication." *ibid.* p. ix.

7. This history explains, for example, the present arrangement of scientific books in university and research libraries using the classification of the Library of Congress, a form of coordination of library resources which has many administrative advantages and is now more widely and strictly adopted than it was before World War II. The scheme for science, developed in the early 1900's, followed rather closely the schedules of the *International Catalogue of Scientific Literature* [Library of Congress, Processing Department, Subject Cataloging Division, *Classification: Class Q, Science* (Government Printing Office, Washington, 5th ed., 1950, reprinted 1957), p. iii]. In spite of some revisions after the first edition of 1905 (2nd ed., 1913; 3rd ed., 1921; 4th ed., 1947), the current schedule reflects basically the state of scientific knowledge as formally structured at the end of the 19th century. As an organizing principle even for the *International Catalogue,* the disciplinary structure had already been challenged in 1896 [C. Adler, "The International Catalogue of Scientific Literature," *Science,* n. s. 6, 184 (1897)]. Aside from the much discussed interdisciplinary and transdisciplinary developments which defy the 19th-century division of subjects, the implicit value judgment as to what constitutes "pure science" no longer applies to current reality, but it still permeates the widely used classification schedule, Class Q. For instance, the schedules of the *International Catalogue* for Human Anatomy, O; for Physiology (including experimental psychology, pharmacology, and experimental pathology), Q; and for Bacteriology, R, are reflected in the Library of Congress schedules QM, Human Anatomy; QP, Physiology (divided into General; Nervous system and the senses, including physiological psychology; Physiological chemistry; and Experimental pharmacology); and QR, Bacteriology (including Immunity and immunization and Viruses). These subjects are in the same class with Mathematics (QA), Astronomy (QB), Geology (QE), etc. They are, however, separated from Class R, Medicine (1st ed., 1910; 2nd ed., 1921; 3rd [rev.] ed., 1952, reprinted 1960); physiological psychology is also separated from the various other classes to which psychology not so identified came to be assigned. Except for the systematic and experimental work considered eligible for the *International Catalogue* in the last few of its 17 schedules, neither medical nor psychological research had achieved the necessary scientific status when those lines were drawn, defining the exact sciences as of 1900. For discussions of some related problems, see the editorial of the *Mental Health Book Review Index* 5, i (January 1960), "The Behavioral sciences and mental health

in relation to the organization of knowledge, the organization of science, and bibliography" [reprinted in *A.M.A. Archives of General Psychiatry* 2, 701 (1960)]; R. C. MacKenzie and Harold Bloomquist, "The impact of the behavioral sciences on the collecting policy of medical school libraries" [2nd Intern. Congr. on Medical Librarianship, Washington, 1963], *Bulletin of the Medical Library Association* 52, 220 (1964).

8. *Bibliographie der deutschen naturwissenschaftlichen Litteratur,* herausgegeben im Auftrage des Reichsamtes des Innern vom Deutschen Bureau der Internationalen Bibliographie in Berlin. 1. Bd., 1901-1902 (Fischer, Jena, 1902), pp. 1258, 1263.

9. W. W. Bishop, "The record of science," *Science* 56, 214 (1922). This statement comes closest to a fundamental critique of the whole undertaking. In the early Twenties the hope persisted that publication of the *International Catalogue* could be resumed on a new basis. Mainly in terms of shortcomings that might be corrected was it acknowledged that the system as originally conceived had broken down. The President of the Royal Society, J. J. Thompson, conceded "that the use that is made of this Catalogue is not so extensive as we had at one time hoped it would be" [Royal Society of London, *Report of the Proceedings at a Conference Called by the Royal Society to Consider the Future of the International Catalogue of Scientific Literature* (London, 1920), p. 11]. By 1922, when the Royal Society withdrew as the responsible publisher, the debts of the *International Catalogue* had reached nearly £12,000 [Royal Society of London, *Yearbook* (1923), pp. 163-164]; only 14 annual issues had been published, covering the years 1901 to 1914; the decennial index, discussed in 1910 [L. C. Gunnell, "The Second International Convention of the International Catalogue of Scientific Literature, London, 1910," *Science* 33, 713 (1911)], was never published so that the set remained without a key. Before publication was to be resumed, the classification schedules were thought to need complete revision "in order to keep abreast with ever advancing discoveries and the consequently changing requirements of investigators and students" [L. C. Gunnell, "Report on the International Catalogue of Scientific Literature," Smithsonian Institution, *Annual Report* (1924), pp. 111-112]. For a noncritical, detailed account with an extensive bibliography, see N. F. Kjösness, *A History of the International Catalogue of Scientific Literature,* master's thesis, Columbia University School of Library Service (1928).

10. H. Carton de Wiart, "Les confins de la littérature et de la science," *Magasin Littéraire* 10, 212 (1893); G. Renard, "La littérature et la science," *Nouvelle Revue* 113, 34 (1898); W. P. Trent, "Litera-

ture and science," address delivered before the Phi Beta Kappa of Lehigh University, 1904, in his *Greatness in Literature and Other Papers* (Crowell, New York, 1905), pp. 109-146; C. L. Morgan, "Science and literature," *Transactions of the Royal Society of Literature,* 2nd ser. 29, 227 (1910); R. E. Rogers, *The Voice of Science in Nineteenth-Century Literature: Representative Prose and Verse* (Atlantic Monthly Press, Boston, 1921); R. A. Scott-James, *The Making of Literature: Some Principles of Criticism Examined in the Light of Ancient and Modern Theory* (Secker, London, 1928; Holt, New York, 1929), pp. 22-24, 336-343; E. De Selincourt, "The interplay of literature and science during the last three centuries," Huxley lecture delivered in the University of Birmingham, 1938, *Hibbert Journal* 37, 225 (1939) [reprinted in his *Wordsworthian and Other Studies* (Clarendon Press, Oxford, 1947), pp. 154-180]; W. L. Bryan, *Wars of Families of Minds,* Powell lectures on philosophy at Indiana University, 4th ser. (Yale Univ. Press, New Haven, 1940), pp. 117-136; G. McColley, Ed., *Literature and Science: an Anthology from English and American Literature, 1600-1900* (Packard, Chicago, 1940), pp. v, 350; H. Eagleson, "The beginning of modern literature," in *Stanford Studies in Language and Literature, 1941,* issued by the School of Letters of Stanford University in honor of the Fiftieth Anniversary of the Founding of Stanford University, H. Craig, Ed., (Stanford Univ. Press, Stanford, 1941), pp. 348-360; H. J. Muller, *Science and Criticism: the Humanistic Tradition in Contemporary Thought* (Yale Univ. Press, New Haven, 1943), p. 267; M. F. Ashley Montagu, "Suggestions for the better correlation of literature and science," in *Studies and Essays in the History of Science and Learning Offered in Homage to George Sarton on the Occasion of His Sixtieth Birthday,* M. F. Ashley Montague, Ed., (Schuman, New York, 1946), pp. 237-246 [contains a list of works, published between 1930 and 1946, illustrating the point that scientific thought, wherever it has flourished, has been reflected in the literature of the day]; F. A. Dudley *et al., The Relations of Literature and Science: a Selected Bibliography, 1930-1949,* published for "General Topics VII," a discussion group of the Modern Language Association of America, by the Department of English of the State College of Washington (State College of Washington, Pullman, 1949); for a continuation of this bibliography by various compilers, see the last of the works cited; B. I. Evans, *Literature and Science* (Allen & Unwin, London, 1954); *Literature and Science* [6th Congress of the International Federation for Modern Languages and Literature, Oxford, 1954], S. C. Aston *et al.,* Eds., (Blackwell, Oxford, 1955); H. Dingle, "The relations between science and literature," *ibid.,* pp. 1-11; C. Day-Lewis, *The Poet's Way of Knowledge,* the Henry Sidgwick memorial lecture, 1956 (Cambridge Univ. Press, Cambridge, England, 1957); H. G. Wood, *Thought, Life and Time as Reflected in Science and Poetry,* the 10th Arthur Stanley Eddington memorial lecture, 1957 (Cambridge Univ. Press, Cambridge, England, 1957); F. E. L. Priestley, " 'Those scattered rays convergent': science and imagination in English literature," in *Science and the Creative Spirit: Essays on Humanistic Aspects of Science,* H. Brown, Ed., (Univ. of Toronto Press, Toronto, 1958), pp. 53-88; A. N. Jeffares, *Language, Literature and Science,* an inaugural lecture, University of Leeds, 1958 (Leeds Univ. Press, Leeds, 1959); E. Sewell, *The Orphic Voice: Poetry and Natural History* (Yale Univ. Press, New Haven, 1960); ——, "Law-courts and dreams," in *The Logic of Personal Knowledge: Essays Presented to Michael Polanyi on His Seventieth Birthday* (Routledge & Paul, London, 1961), pp. 179-188; E. C. Blunden, *English Scientists as Men of Letters,* Jubilee Congress lecture, University of Hong Kong, 1961 (Univ. of Hong Kong Press, Hong Kong; Oxford Univ. Press, New York, London, 1961); A. Huxley, *Literature and Science* (Harper & Row, New York; Chatto & Windus, London, 1963); N. Kiell, "Criticism, literary, psychoanalytic, psychological," in his *Psychoanalysis, Psychology, and Literature: a Bibliography* (Univ. of Wisconsin Press, Madison, 1963), pp. 32-57. For further references, see the annual selected bibliography, "Relations of literature and science," published on behalf of General Topics VII (Literature and Science) of the Modern Language Association in *Symposium: a Quarterly Journal in Modern Literatures* 5 (1951) to date (slightly irregular).

11. J. M. Drachman, *Studies in the Literature of Natural Science,* thesis, Columbia University (Macmillan, New York, 1930); G. McColley, Ed., *Literature and Science: an Anthology from English and American Literature, 1600-1900* (Packard, Chicago, 1940), p. 4; M. Cowley and B. Smith, Eds., *Books That Changed Our Minds* (Doubleday, Doran, New York, 1939, 1940); R. B. Downs, *Books That Changed the World* (American Library Association, Chicago, 1956); ——, *Molders of the Modern Mind: 111 Books That Shaped Western Civilization* (Barnes & Noble, New York, 1961).

12. Recent bibliographic developments concerned with Festschriften may serve to illustrate this point. An attempt to note Festschriften in a branch of science was made in the *Bibliography and Index of Geology Exclusive of North America,* M. Siegrist, Mary C. Grier *et al.,* Eds., (Geological Society of America, New York), which from vol. 22, 1957 (1958) to vol. 26, 1961 (1963) has listed 39 publications under the special heading "Festschrifts" (vol. 22, p. xv; vol. 23, p. xvii; vol. 24, p. xviii; vol. 25, p. xvi; vol. 26, p. xvi). For a list of 8 indexes to Festschriften

mainly in the humanities, of which 6 were published since 1951, see D. Rounds, *Articles on Antiquity in Festschriften, an Index: the Ancient Near East, the Old Testament, Greece, Rome, Roman Law, Byzantium* (Harvard Univ. Press, Cambridge, 1962), p. 553. This work includes also the first comprehensive paper on the subject, D. Rounds and S. Dow, "Festschriften," (pp. 551-560), originally published in *Harvard Library Bulletin* 8, 283 (1954). Completing the cooperative work of 25 countries, which had been interrupted by World War II, the International Committee of Historical Sciences published its *Bibliographie internationale des travaux historiques publiés dans les volumes de "mélanges," 1880-1939* (Colin, Paris, 1955). In 1958 the Foreign Law Committee of the American Association of Law Libraries, Kurt Schwerin, chairman, gave special recognition to Festschriften in law, which have since been studied and are now indexed in various current legal bibliographies; see L. M. Roberts, "The importance of legal Festschriften for work in international and comparative law," *American Journal of Comparative Law* 11, 403 (1962); ——, "Legal Festschriften," *Law Library Journal* 56, 47 (1963), with an annotated list of 12 Festschriften bibliographies which include legal material; three of these, confined to law, were published since 1956. An index to Festschriften dealing with 'Germanistik,' based on the collections of the University of London, was proposed in 1959; see R. Pick, "Some thoughts on Festschriften and a projected subject index," *German Life and Letters* 12, 204 (1959). Additional recent indexes to Festschriften are: G. Thils, *Theologica et Miscellaneis* (Warny, Louvain, 1960); P. O. Rave and B. Stein, *Kunstgeschichte in Festschriften: Allgemeine Bibliographie kunstwissenschaftlicher Abhandlungen in den bis 1960 erschienenen Festschriften* (Mann, Berlin, 1962). Between 1951 and 1962, 13 indexes to Festschriften appeared in major areas of scholarship, which analyze from a few hundred to nearly 1,500 volumes in their respective fields. It would be a mistake to conclude from the lack of comparable studies and bibliographies of Festschriften in science that these are not numerous or important enough. Rather, the emphasis on computer-oriented current information services tends to conceal developments in the literature of science which, in other areas, have been revealed by advances in scholarly bibliography. This poses the question whether scientific bibliography, geared to recency of information, may not have fallen behind in the observation of new trends and the planning of newly conceived projects.

13. Preoccupation with the rising number of scientific publications has obscured the fact that publishing activities are closely related to the size of the reading public and do not reflect a corresponding gain in sub-

stance. For a broader historical perspective on the effect of education and mass education on literary output over a wide range of quality, see J. W. Thompson, *The Literacy of the Laity in the Middle Ages* (Univ. of California Press, Berkeley, 1939); A. S. Collins, *Authorship in the Days of Johnson, Being a Study of the Relation between Author, Patron, Publisher and Public, 1726-1780* (Holden, London, 1927), pp. 213-270; ——, *The Profession of Letters: a Study of the Relation of Author to Patron, Publisher, and Public, 1780-1832* (Routledge, London, 1928); A. M. Schlesinger, "American history and American literary history," in *The Reinterpretation of American Literature: Some Contributions Toward the Understanding of Its Historical Development,* N. Foerster, Ed., (Harcourt, Brace, New York, 1928; Russell, New York, 1959), pp. 160-180; F. W. Halsey, *Our Literary Deluge and Some of Its Deeper Waters* (Doubleday, Page, New York, 1902), pp. 3-8; H. Sullivan, "Literacy and illiteracy," in *Encyclopedia of the Social Sciences,* vol. 9, pp. 511-523. For suggestions of an inverse relationship between quantity of information and quality of knowledge, see also P. Weiss, "Knowledge: a growth process," *Science* 131, 1716 (1960) [printed simultaneously in *Proceedings of the American Philosophical Society* 104, 242 (1960)]; V. M. Pings, "The specter of automated creativity," *College and Research Libraries* 24, 119 (1963); P. A. Richmond, "What are we looking for?", *Science* 139, 737 (1963); P. H. Abelson, Editorial: "Information transfer and retrieval," *Science* 141, 319 (1963).

14. A large body of critical writing concerned with forms, problems, and standards of scientific literature exists, but is now submerged. It can be found in introductions to, and reviews of, certain types of scientific publication, e.g., conferences and symposia, readers and anthologies, handbooks and encyclopedias, Festschriften and other collections. The neglect of these forms of publication in the prevailing pattern of scientific bibliography tends to suppress this criticism, through which the scientists themselves contribute to the formation and articulation of scientific literature, thus repeating an earlier phase in the relationship between writer and critic; cf. R. A. Scott-James, who points out that the world's most remarkable literary critics include Aristophanes, Horace, Dante, Ben Jonson, Dryden, Goethe, Coleridge, and Matthew Arnold [*The Making of Literature: Some Principles of Criticism Examined in the Light of Ancient and Modern Theory* (Secker, London, 1928; Holt, New York, 1929), p. 14]. For examples of applying different techniques of literary criticism to scientific literature and modes of scientific discourse, see G. Temple, "Style and subject in the literature of mathematics," in *Literature and Science* [6th Congr. of the Intern. Federation for Modern Languages and Literature, Oxford, 1954], S. C. Aston *et al.*,

Eds., (Blackwell, Oxford, 1955), pp. 11-16; A. Rapoport, "The language of science: its simplicity, beauty, and humor," *ETC.: a Review of General Semantics* 16, 445 (1959).

15. For an exposition of the complex problems involved in the major aspects of book reviews, see M. M. Kinney, M. Franck, I. Bry, "The book review—a hybrid in literature and a stepchild in documentation," in *International Congress of Libraries and Documentation Centres,* Brussels, 1955 (Nijhoff, The Hague, 1955), vol. IIA, pp. 80-86.

16. For an analysis of data about 20,000 reviews of almost 9,000 books and pamphlets reviewed in at least one of 150 journals in the English language relating to the behavioral sciences and the mental health professions and indexed for 6 years (1955-1961), see the editorial, "Book reviewing in the sciences of human behavior as a contribution to scholarship by the scientific community," *Mental Health Book Review Index* 6, i (1961). About half of the reviews were concentrated on some 2,000 books; 7,000 of the reviews could be traced to 18 journals in psychology, psychiatry, and psychoanalysis, 13,000 were scattered through 130 journals, including all the recent and multidisciplinary journals covered. For illustrations of the selection achieved by the "invisible panel of judges" formed by the editors, book review editors, and reviewers of the journals which contribute to this collective process, see also the editorial, "The conservation of knowledge about human behavior," *Mental Health Book Review Index* 7, i (1962). An interesting beginning toward the collating of book reviews in a single discipline in science has been made in recent years by the Documentation Research Project of the American Institute of Physics; see especially its *Annual Physics Book List—1962: a Compilation of the 1962 "Books Received" Listings in Physics Today with Review Citations from Six Leading Physics Journals* (1963).

17. Quoted in L. P. Betz, *Studien zur vergleichenden Literaturgeschichte der neueren Zeit* (Rütten & Loening, Frankfurt a. M., 1902), p. 13.

18. R. A. Scott-James, *The Making of Literature: Some Principles of Criticism Examined in the Light of Ancient and Modern Theory* (Secker, London, 1928; Holt, New York, 1929), p. 14.

19. J. Maddox, "Is the literature worth keeping?" *Rockefeller Institute Review* 1, 9 (February 1963); an abridged version appears in *Bulletin of the Atomic Scientists* 19, 14 (November 1963). An example of the ambiguity of the term *scientific literature* in current usage is the *Bibliography of Publications Designed to Raise the Standard of Scientific Literature* (UNESCO, Paris, 1963), which uses the following more descriptive headings for its 359 entries: 1) General works on lan-

guage and composition; 2) The technique of technical writing; 3) Books on editing, printing and publishing; 4) Information retrieval and indexing; 5) Readings in science for technical authors; and 6) Handbooks for authors.

20. Plans for creating a nationwide automated library system for the large research libraries, to be based on automation of the Library of Congress, throw new light on the fact that the projected technology could be most constructively applied to bibliographic data more highly developed than those now available and significant enough, not only numerous enough, to be a match for the computer. To obtain such data is not an engineering problem but depends on corresponding advances in bibliographic theory and concepts; see G. W. King *et al.*, *Automation and the Library of Congress: a Survey Sponsored by the Council on Library Resources, Inc.* (Library of Congress, Washington, 1963 [i.e. 1964]); J. Walsh, "Library of Congress automation urged for bibliographic control but not prescribed as a panacea," *Science* 143, 452 (1964). For a historical perspective on the efforts to achieve bibliographic control in medicine, from the early 16th to the mid-20th century, see E. Brodman, *The Development of Medical Bibliography*, thesis, Columbia University (Medical Library Association [Waverly Press, Baltimore], 1954).

# ESSAY 7

## *Bibliographical Challenges in the Age of the Computer*

Originally published as Editorial in *Mental Health Book Review Index,* vol. 9 (whole no. 14), 1964. Reprinted here from an edited version published in *Library Journal,* vol. 90, no. 4, February 15, 1965, pp. 813-818.

The prediction that automation will free us from drudgery for more imaginative and creative work has come to be more soberly understood as implying that our imagination and creativity must stay ahead of the expanding capability of the computer. In bibliography, we have to be ready for the new ways in which computers stand ready to assist us. The question posed by advancing automation is not, what is the challenge of utilizing computers, but rather, what are the new challenges to bibliography today? We shall suggest what we see as three immediate bibliographical challenges, illustrating them with observations drawn from our own work in the behavioral sciences, but hoping also to draw attention to some broader problems in the bibliography of science and scholarship.

"On the Difficulty of Correct Description of Books" is the title of an essay by the mathematician and bibliographer August de Morgan, published in 1853, with the intention "to show, by instances, to how great an extent inaccurate bibliography prevails, both in the descriptions which are given of books, and in those which they give of themselves." In the mid-19th Century, the British Government sought to deal with the rising need for bibliographic and library services to scientists and the public, much as Congressional committees in the United States have done in the early 1960's. Before a Royal Commission, appointed to examine the state of the British Museum, de Morgan testified in favor of giving full titles in the Library's Catalogue. He predicted that, if entries were shortened, this would tend to perpetuate the already abundant errors and, in subsequent use, give rise to more and more errors.

## TITLE-PAGE VAGARIES

In de Morgan's time, it was understood that a book was reasonably well described by a full transcript of its title-page. Since then, and especially in the behavioral sciences, the title-page has become a poor medium for bibliographic communication. Books in these fields now reach multiple audiences. Quite often the title-page is designed to stimulate the interest of the largest possible public, and the information given tends to be vague and open to diverse interpretations, approaching the simplified message of the book jacket, now frankly a medium of book promotion. The more complicated data, which might earlier have been put in a subtitle, are relegated to prefaces, acknowledgments, introductions, or epilogues.

For illustrations, we invite readers who might want to form their own judgment to look at the entries reproduced here from the *Mental Health Book Review Index* which contain information in brackets (Fig. 1). This portion of the "correct description of books" does not appear on the title-page. These data may be irrelevant for the lay reader and might even deter him. Scientists and scholars, however, with their limited time, need the salient facts, directly and clearly stated. Without having to seek out the book, scientists would want to know, for example, whether it is a report of research or of a conference and, if so, what kind, with the dates and chief delimitations, the auspices and contributors. Types of data that often have to be added are: significant aspects of subject matter or scope which cannot be inferred from the title; antecedents such as prior publication; and for translations, title and date of the original.

Sometimes the very particulars which would serve to characterize a specific book are missing from the title-page, for instance, that a book on schizophrenia contains a survey and extensive bibliography of the pertinent Russian literature (Fig. 1); and that a *Tribute to Freud,* while first appearing in book form in 1956, was not one of many eulogies

2694. Astrup, Christian. Schizophrenia; conditional reflex studies. [A report of research and a survey of Russian studies of the higher nervous activity in mental disorders, with extensive bibliography. With an index of Russian journals and congress reports.] Foreword by W. Horsley Gantt. Springfield, Ill., Thomas, 1962. 345 p. (American lecture series, publ. no. 471. American lectures in objective psychiatry) 13.75

2752. Doolittle, Hilda. Tribute to Freud, by H.D. With unpublished letters by Freud to the author. [An account of Hilda Doolittle Aldington's psychoanalysis with Freud, originally publ. with title Writing on the wall: to Sigmund Freud, blameless physician, in Life and Letters To-day, vol. 45, May and June, 1945, p. 67-98, 137-154; vol. 46, August and September, 1945, p. 72-89, 136-151; vol. 48, January 1946, p. 33-45.] Foreword by Merrill Moore. N.Y., Pantheon, 1956, 180 p. 2.50

Fig. 1: The fact that the bracketed bibliographic data do not appear on the title-page raises questions about the practice and purpose of descriptive bibliography.

written for the centenary of Freud's birth, but is the account of Hilda Doolittle's psychoanalysis with Freud, serially published a decade earlier in a British magazine (Fig. 1). There is a chain effect here. When such particulars are overlooked in the first round of bibliographic descriptions, the book may later be missed by the compilers of more specialized bibliographies and reference works, as has happened in some such instances. The loss to the scientific community then becomes increasingly severe.

Ad hoc measures, to some extent, make up for the damage to scholarship. The book trade reaches scientists through judicious advertising, book clubs, exhibits at scientific conventions, and so forth. Some scholarly-minded reviewers now make it their business to state first of all what a book is, besides what it purports to be. In academic and research libraries, professional catalogers may boil down the essentials into a note, when administrative conditions permit. Spontaneous, scattered bibliographic descriptions are, however, not channeled into the organized bibliographic record.

Our first bibliographical challenge, then, is to subject descriptive bibliography to a thorough revision and reconstruction in the light of social and scientific changes, in order to be able to profit from the gains made by technological changes. Our bibliographic style first has to be raised again to the level of scholarly communication. Then we can undertake to restore, under contemporary conditions, the true purpose of bibliography, which is today, as it has been in the past, to arrive at a record of knowledge and thus serve its continuity, dissemination, and advancement. How to approach this goal is a question that involves more fundamental issues, to which we will now turn.

In "Evidence and Inference in Bibliography," a paper given at the third English Institute at Columbia University in 1941, R. C. Bald pointed out that, although we might conceivably be able to reproduce a 17th-Century printing house down to the last detail, "the making of books is a human activity, and the human factor is the incalculable with which we must always reckon." Nothing has ever forced this fact as strongly upon our awareness as the advent of the computer. And no other single human factor may be as crucial here as the proper balance of evidence and inference.

To draw inferences is indeed, as Shakespeare knew and John Stuart Mill spelled out, "the great business of life." The role of inference in human relations and communication, in our thinking and activities, is now being studied in many fields. In bibliography, we have barely begun to face the issue, although it is here of paramount importance. Traditionally, scholarly bibliography has aimed at creating a system that allows us to draw from a minimum of words a maximum of correct, significant inferences.

The bibliographic code is not in itself the evidence that supports our inferences; it only stands for a certain type of evidence and is useful only as long as that evidence remains unchanged. To take a very simple example: in the current volume of the *Index,* one review citation gives the pages, "126-132." In the scientific literature, this usually implies that the review is seven pages long, and the book presumably an important one. In this instance, however, it is supposed to imply merely that the review begins on p. 126 and ends on p. 132; in between, the review takes up three columns, whereas ten columns are filled with advertisements. Since we are now aware of the continuous change in matters that have a bearing upon the bibliographic code, one of the challenges to bibliography today is to provide a basis for inferences which will remain valid in spite of such changes.

For this purpose, we will have to gather evidence about the "making" of scientific and scholarly books today, not in the physical sense, which is now incidental, but as an intellectual and social process. In the early days, the author's relationships with his patron and his printer may have seemed complicated enough. Now we have instead several vast systems, all differently organized and only partially relating to one another.

## COMPLEX OF COMMUNITIES

There is first the scientific community, where the book originates. It is represented by authors, editors, and scientists in various supporting roles. Then there is the now exceedingly complex network of sponsoring bodies, which lend their auspices, give financial support, or do both. This system encompasses universities and scientific societies, government, industry, large or small foundations, and the innumerable organizations serving special causes. Those responsible for publishing form the third system. It partly overlaps with the second system, and its scholarly participation, through its power of selection, extends farther than is generally realized. By international arrangements and the distribution of book review copies, publishers are often able to speed the first scholarly recognition of the book. The scientific community then enters once more into the picture; with an enormous, completely unstructured and thus most flexible and functional network of interrelated competencies, it now directs itself to the evaluation of the literature and the gradual crystallization of knowledge. Many scientists serve concurrently in several capacities, as authors, editors, reviewers within the scientific community, in their respective affiliations with the "sponsoring community," and as consultants to publishers.

All these systems interact in providing the background for the emerging literature. The systems themselves cannot be coordinated or required to produce one type of data in a form suitable for bibliographic processing. To unify the diverse data is the task of bibliography. It has been customary to account for two of the four systems in our bibliographic entries, by indicating author and publisher. In order to do justice to the more complex nature of the contemporary scientific literature, we also have to give some representation to the other two systems. This is what we have been trying to do in the *Index*. In our List of Journals Indexed, and where called for in the entries for the books, we show the sponsoring bodies that are involved in one way or another.

And we give a continuous record of the critical reviews, with the comments and controversies they elicit, after a certain accumulation of reviews begins to suggest that a collective evaluation is under way.

When all bibliographic data point in the same direction, as in the case of a standard textbook, there is no problem. The risk of drawing false inferences enters when the impression of a simple situation is given, although the facts are really more complex. In our presentation this would become apparent through a conflict in the bibliographic data. For example, in the context of elaborate research, a title that may suggest a work of fiction will not be so interpreted; a reference to a review of an older book in a recent scholarly journal may convey that the work is still intellectually valid; when a nonprofit organization acts as publisher, a smaller number of reviews can carry more weight; and when a book review stirs up an unusual type of controversy, this might point up other problems, e.g., those involved in industry-sponsored efforts to disseminate information.

## COMPUTERS AND OBSOLESCENCE

After we have learned to determine what evidence concerning the nature of the book is essential and must be retained in the bibliographic presentation, we might consider the use of computers for the storage and further analysis of appropriately prepared data. If, however, the data have been stored in such a way that part of the essential evidence has dropped out of the picture and has been replaced by bibliographic symbols and clues that will become obsolete, such as subject headings or classification codes, the accuracy of inferences to be drawn is bound to diminish. The question then arises, on what scale might we be able to afford a programming of computers so that the data stored hold a maximum of the necessary evidence in support of permanently sound inferences? This raises the issue of selection.

In the preface to his William James lectures, *The Place of Value in a World of Facts,* given at Harvard in 1934 and published in 1938, Wolfgang Köhler referred to the serious doubts that had then been raised "as to whether, in its present course, science will be able to contribute much to the fundamental issues of mankind." This concern deepened in the decade that followed and helped the behavioral sciences to crystallize.

## SOMETHING OF VALUE

To find "the place of value in a world of facts" presents a third, and the greatest, challenge to bibliography in the age of the computer. The need to evaluate the literature before storing it is now generally granted. The bibliographic services developed by the scientific community in the 19th Century were selective, and this tradition continues in the more specialized annual reviews. As a reaction to the non-selective information services, there has been a strong demand for more reviewing and evaluating of the literature, but the mass of publications to be surveyed makes this task increasingly hopeless. One possible new approach would be to base selection on the pooling of competent evaluations already made.

The scientific community is implicitly engaged in a continuous process of creating, recognizing, and rewarding values. At all times, some of its members are specifically concerned with excellence and distinction: they propose and judge prize essays, invite distinguished scientists to give endowed lectures, make the selections for scientific awards and the arrangements for special honors and tributes. Much of this evaluative process leaves a mark in the literature and is then open to further evaluation. As yet, scanty provisions have been made for transcribing such marks of distinction in bibliographic records, with an emphasis on the initial evaluation.

The appropriate contemporaneous sources report scholarly honors, e.g., in the news notes of journals or as biographical data. A wealth of such information exists. A computer could store these data and be programmed to tell which scientists were distinguished or rewarded, for which contributions under what auspices, and with what results in published form. A bibliography of these publications on a universal scale, not merely limited to the widely publicized Nobel prizes, might get us far in mapping out the major research and ideological advances of our time.

## EDITORIAL EVALUATIONS

Furthermore, editors express value judgments not only by accepting or rejecting manuscripts. They add "value accents," through position

**2911.** Riese, Hertha Pataky. Heal the hurt child; an approach through educational therapy with special reference to the extremely deprived Negro child. [Presentation of a method developed at the Educational Therapy Center in Richmond, Virginia.] Foreword by Nathan W. Ackerman. Chicago, London, Univ. of Chicago Pr., 1962. 615 p. 10.00; 72s

Arch. gen. Psychiat., 1963,
9, 103 (Eugene I. Falstein)
Bull. Inst. Child Study, 1963,
25 (1), 15 (Karl S. Bernhardt)
Bull. Menninger Clin., 1964,
28, 93 (Edwin Z. Levy)
Canad. psychiat. Ass. J., 1963,
8, 354-355 (R.J. McQueen)
Child Welf., 1963,
42, 508-509 (Saul Hofstein)
Contemp. Psychol., 1963,
8, 433-434 (Wilbert W. Lewis)
Fed. Probation, 1963,
27 (4), 71-72 (John B. Thomas)
Int. J. Group Psychother., 1963,
13, 497-498 (Beatrice Liebenberg)
Ment. Hosp., 1963,
14, 299-300 (Harry G. Moore, Jr.)
Psychol. Rec., 1963,
13, 517 (Emma Layman)
Social Serv. Rev., 1963,
37, 223-224 (Robert Kohrman)
Social Wk, N.Y., 1963,
8 (4), 117-118 (Nancy Staver)

Fig. 2: Emphasis on social responsibility in science brings out the involvement of various scientific and professional groups, as reflected in the sources of the cited reviews.

in a journal, the space allowed, editorial comments, or a distinctive form of presentation, such as the "critical notice" reserved in some British journals for significant works. Scientists who read or scan the journals note the signs of the editors' evaluations, but these are disregarded in the process of indexing and thus are not shown in the secondary records. By retaining the tokens of recognition already achieved, we could make our bibliographic presentation more articulate. Moreover, it is fundamental to both the scientific and the democratic process that the value system underlying the advancement of science should be as highly visible as possible. Only then can it be continually and effectively reassessed.

Although the method we are developing in the *Index* is a small beginning, we may venture to suggest how the emerging fusion of values and facts might be made visible with bibliographic means. The books reviewed in journals from many fields and with great earnestness and concern are often those with an explicit emphasis on the social aspects of the subject. Social responsibility in science, long regarded as a matter of the scientist's personal ethics, has become an integral part of much of the work undertaken within, or sanctioned by, the behavioral sciences. This is reflected, for example, in the book entitled *Heal the Hurt Child; an Approach through Educational Therapy with Special Reference to the Extremely Deprived Negro Child* (Fig. 2). Books on such topics as

**2892.** Osgood, Charles Egerton. An alternative to war or surrender. Urbana, Ill., Univ. of Illinois Pr., 1962, 183 p. (Illini books, IB-7) 1.45

Amer. J. Orthopsychiat., 1963, 33, 183-191 (Milton Schwebel & Murray Krim: Human survival: a selected bibliography)

Brit. J. Psychol., 1963, 54, 188-189 (T.H. Pear)

J. Confl. Resol., 1963, 7, 141-149 (Fred A. Sondermann: Peace initiatives; the literature of possibilities)

Social Probl., 1963/64, 11, 106-116 (Michael Maccoby: Social scientists on war and peace: an essay-review)

Fig. 3: Through the citing of essay reviews, the listing of one book can become the key to the bibliography of an emerging subject.

human survival, creativity, and computer applications in the behavioral sciences, tend to be recognized and brought together in essay reviews and critical annotated bibliographies. Our review citations then become early "bibliographies of bibliographies" on the pioneer work (Fig. 3). Some of the essay titles may also convey the nature of the concern, e.g., "Teaching Behavioral Scientists How to Use Their Brains," or "Peace Initiatives: the Literature of Possibilities."

Thus, while making the language of bibliography ready for the computer, we must make the conceptual framework of bibliography ready for a science that has set its course so that it may "be able to contribute much to the fundamental issues of mankind." What we need first are pioneers, people who do what has to be done "lovingly, not drudgingly," without asking what in their work is delight, what dedication, and what drudgery. Indeed, as automation advances, we must watch out: it may claim as drudgery and take off our hands the work-a-day experience that may trigger the imagination and creativity for which we are supposed to be freed.

Intellectual discipline sometimes looks like routine. In the age of the computer, the danger of confusing the qualities that make the difference has taken on new dimensions, but in essence the problem has been recognized before. In 1755, Samuel Johnson put it as a joke turned on himself, by defining a lexicographer as "a harmless drudge, that busies himself in tracing the original, and detailing the signification of words." A century later, the joke had become a taunt. In his essay of 1853, August de Morgan quoted the reviewer of a catalog of Cardinal Mezzofanti's library, made by a Roman bookseller, who entered a Cingalese grammar, printed at Colombo, under the United States of America: "It may help to enforce a truism which seems of late years to have been almost entirely lost sight of . . . that the making of catalogues correctly, like the making of dictionaries, requires in the 'harmless drudge' who practices it an amount of qualifications which those who despise him are often far from possessing." Today this is no longer a truism, but it is still true.

# ESSAY 8

## *In Search of an Organizing Principle for the Behavioral Science Literature*

Originally published as Editorial in *Mental Health Book Review Index,* vol. 10 (whole no. 15), 1965. Reprinted here in an adapted version with references from *Community Mental Health Journal,* vol. 4, no. 1, February 1968, pp. 75-84.

With the growth and acceptance of the behavioral sciences it has become important to distinguish the behavioral science literature from the other literature concerned with man and the innumerable expressions of human life. Publications resulting from the scientific study of human behavior are available in libraries and recorded in general bibliographies. They have not, however, been identified and brought together as relating to one new scientific field.

The problem of bibliographic organization extends to the mental health literature when *mental health* is defined as a field that "makes use of a core of knowledge, contributed by the behavioral sciences, and amplifies it with scientific, professional, and social ramifications and applications" (Editorial, 1960, p. 703). As community mental health becomes a new force in study, teaching, and social action, it stimulates concern for more adequate access to the literature. Public libraries and, increasingly, college and university libraries, are cultural centers of the community and, therefore, share this concern. When mental health and library services are both community oriented, demands for the literature on human behavior expand in new directions, and there is a new need to understand the conditions under which this literature is organized. The complex issues involved may become clearer when they are considered in the light of the history of ideas.

## THE SCIENCES OF MAN

The most widely used systems of bibliographic and library classification were influenced by the ideology prevailing in the latter part of the 19th century. The period from 1830 to 1890 had brought large technological and social changes. The philosophical concern with man as a whole was then declining, while the search for truth and knowledge was shifting to the special disciplines. In a recent proposal to regroup the classes of the decimal classification scheme, Raoul Dubuc (1963), a French documentalist, pointed out that, although most of the classes of the Dewey and the Universal Decimal Classifications relate to man, it had not occurred to the founders of these classifications to create a focus for the "sciences of man." Nor had there been any general concern about that in the last quarter of the 19th century.

The concept "sciences of man," already known in the 16th century, was elaborated in the romantic period which encouraged a deep interest in human nature. Philosophers, physicians, novelists, and poets sought insight into phenomena such as the unconscious, dreams, and mental illness, which behavioral scientists now study with more rigorous methods. In various philosophical encylopedic systems of knowledge, devised in the late 18th and early 19th centuries, the terms "anthropological sciences," "human sciences," and "sciences of man" were used interchangeably (Petzholdt, 1866). The author of one of these systems, first published in 1796, was Wilhelm Traugott Krug, Kant's successor as professor of philosophy. Krug's anthropological sciences comprise the study of man's body (Somatology) and mind (Psychology) and of man as a whole (Anthropology), as an individual and in social relationships (Political Sciences).

One hundred years later, Edmond Goblot, who then became professor of the history of philosophy and science at the University of Lyons, modified the philosophical concept of the study of man in the light of the scientific progress made during the 19th century. Goblot was remarkably free from the thinking in narrow disciplinary terms so often found at that time. In his thesis *Essai sur la Classification des Sciences* of 1898, he insisted that the study of living organisms must encompass all manifestations of life–physiological, psychological, and sociological–and must unite the study of the individual and the group. He combined the pertinent sciences in one table with the heading, *Bio-*

*Psycho-Sociologie.* The table included physiology, biology, geography, history, and the medical sciences, with subdivisions for the organic, psychological, and social aspects under various main categories. It should be noted that psychology did not appear as an independent main category, but rather as a catalyst or a link between the organic and social functions of living organisms: plants, animals, and men.

Another half century elapsed before the anthropological or human sciences and the concept of bio-psycho-sociology were introduced into library classification and documentation. Henry E. Bliss (1952-53), an American librarian, brought the ideas of the romantic period to bear upon his effort to systematize the literature of 20th-century science. Like Goblot, Bliss proposed that the biological, psychological, and social sciences be regarded not as strictly isolated classes, but rather as classes characterized by subject matter and problems biological, mental, and social. However, the closest he could come to adopting this idea in his own classification was to place the human sciences in a contiguous sequence. The Bliss Classification appeared in 1952. One year later, Eric de Grolier (1953), professor at the Institut National des Techniques de Documentation in Paris, proposed a new encyclopedic scheme that also contains the concepts, "bio-psycho-sociology" and "Human Sciences, Anthropology." The latter begin with man, physical and mental, in a group joining together human biology, medicine, human psychology, and ethnology, and continue through the social sciences to the humanities.

About 1950, American scientists introduced the name "behavioral sciences" as a term equally acceptable to specialists in the psychological, biological, and social sciences (Miller, 1955; Senn, 1966). In the fullest early definition published, Roy R. Grinker (1953, p. 189), editor of the journal *Archives of General Psychiatry,* explained that behavioral science

> deals with man as a biological organism striving as part of his animal, human, and physical environment for continuity and for self-fulfillment as an individual, as he integrates into varying-sized groups.

A spokesman for those willing to identify themselves with the behavioral sciences at that early stage has been the editor of the journal *Behavioral Science,* James G. Miller, professor of psychiatry and psychology and director of the Mental Health Research Institute at the University of Michigan.

Although leading librarians and documentalists had by that time laid the groundwork for a corresponding orientation in international bibliography, the relevance of these parallel trends to each other was not recognized. With few exceptions (MacKenzie and Bloomquist, 1964), the impact on the library field so far has been limited to intellectual interest without practical consequences. In this country, virtually all university, college, and public libraries use the established Library of Congress or the Dewey classifications, which have become an intrinsic part of the American library system. In spite of earlier opposition, these two schemes seem to be gaining also in libraries abroad. Their advantages could apply to the behavioral sciences, if a supplementary bibliographic system were available. In the classifications rooted in the 19th century, as they are used now, "man as a whole" and as part of a more complex social organism has been thoroughly dismembered. In fact, man does not really appear as the object of knowledge at all.

## MAN–EXPLORING OR EXPLORED

Although lacking the concept of "human sciences," the encyclopedic systems which influenced the leading library classifications were also concerned with man. Man was seen as being in the center of the search for knowledge, and the fields of knowledge were grouped according to an imaginary sequence in this pursuit. Such systems may be called anthropocentric. The reasoning said to underlie the Dewey Decimal Classification (Coulson, 1911) follows this anthropocentric pattern: After man has formed the concept of existence (Philosophy, 100), he tries to regulate his relations with the Creator of his existence (Religion, 200) and organizes his society (Sociology, 300), where men use language (Philology, 400) to exchange ideas about their discoveries in Natural Science (500). The use of objects simplifies man's existence (Useful Arts, 600). Man then has the leisure to beautify his surroundings (Fine Arts, 700). Finally, he puts his ideas into Literature (800) and undertakes to record all preserved knowledge in History (900). This rationale explains, among other things, the separation of language from literature, which has been so impractical for modern libraries.

We may coin the word "anthropotropic" for systems that reflect the "turning toward man" in man's search for knowledge about himself.

The possible transition from an anthropocentric to an anthropotropic approach is suggested in a system published in 1798 by A. G. Camus, the organizer of the French Archives Nationales, as a contribution to library classification (Petzholdt, 1866). He, too, wanted to arrange the subject fields in the order in which they presumably present themselves to a man untouched by civilization and eager to learn. Camus' natural man first surveys the wonders of the whole universe, but then he returns to his own person in order to study himself, to perfect himself, to measure the extent of knowledge of which he is capable. From the study of the nature of man, of education and the formation of languages, he turns to the sciences and arts, probes into the bases of society, and arrives at the various social studies.

The positivistic school of thought of the 19th century had much in common with this outlook, except for the reflection upon man himself which later became the essence of the behavioral sciences. In Comte's final classification of knowledge, published in 1854, Mathematics, Astronomy, Physics, Chemistry, Biology, Sociology, and Morality follow one another. The order is supposed to lead from the simpler to the more complex and has been said to reflect an evolutionary mode of thinking. Comte denied in his system of the sciences a place to psychology. He did much, however, to direct attention to the social aspects of life and, in this respect, greatly influenced later classifications of books, including that of Melvil Dewey.

Inevitably, classification schemes that are completely anthropocentric must be inhospitable to the literature of the behavioral sciences which, by definition, are anthropotropic. This dilemma has not gone unnoticed. When man's search for knowledge about himself was profoundly changed by the advent of psychology as a science, the question arose of finding a place for the new field.

## MAN'S SELF-EXPLORATION AS A SCIENCE

Three problems stand out in the recurrent discussions of that question. The first problem concerns the conceptual framework that underlies the treatment of psychology in library classifications. The rise of psychology as an autonomous discipline occurred during the last quarter of the 19th century. It thus paralleled the rise of professional library organization in which a standardized subject approach to books played a major part. Most of the work done at the frontiers of the new science was scattered in the existing nonpsychological journals. It was not yet clearly enough identified with a new discipline to serve as a basis for representing modern psychology in the Dewey Decimal and the Library of Congress classifications of books. The philosophical background rather than the scientific perspectives provided the primary pattern for classifying psychology in libraries. Although the Dewey Classification was repeatedly revised, no attempt was made to change its basic structure.

In 1931, the American Psychological Association (1931, p. 656) officially informed the Library of Congress of its belief that the Library's

> classification for psychology is antiquated and confused, and that it neither represents the present articulation of the subject nor the external relations of psychology to many related sciences and arts.

However, nothing came of the Association's offer to assist the Library of Congress in a reconstruction of psychological topics which would be of very great service to psychological users of libraries and "would much more intelligently represent to the general reading public the present status, methods, and accomplishments of psychology." Howard C. Warren (1931), a past president of the American Psychological Association who had been editor of the *Psychological Index* from its start in 1894 for almost 20 years, made this appraisal of the Dewey system:

> It is based on pre-Wundtian and pre-Jamesian conceptions. A few of the topics are scientifically elaborated; but most of the newer departments are treated in a fragmentary way, and related topics are so scattered about that no contemporary psychologist could utilize the schema in his work. On the other hand, all branches of pseudopsychology and magic are worked out more than adequately. It would probably have suited Thomas Aquinas and other medieval psychologists admirably.

The second problem concerns the scientific relationship between psychology and psychiatry. During the first half of the 20th century, these two disciplines converged toward unity of knowledge. As president of the First World Congress of Psychiatry held in Paris in 1950, Jean Delay

(1956), professor of psychiatry and director of the Institut de Psychologie at the Sorbonne, summarized the development that had led to modern psychiatry. He called the physiological and psychological approaches dissimilar but indissoluble and likened them to a Janus who would become meaningless if the two faces were separated. During the past 15 years, the integration of psychology, psychiatry, and psychoanalysis has progressed in research and higher education, in symposia, books, and journals, but hardly in bibliography. Their separation, which perpetuates an old pattern of scientific organization, is firmly built into the leading library classifications. Attempted adjustments, such as the transfer of clinical psychology and parts of psychoanalysis from the psychological to the medical schedules, have only added to the difficulties. The old division persists also in general bibliographic sources such as the national bibliographies of Canada, England, France, Germany, India, Russia, and many other countries, all of which use a classified scheme. Through constant reinforcement within a worldwide bibliographic machinery, the separation by disciplines greatly interferes with recognition of progress in the psychological sciences. The only major bibliographic system that has a single class for psychology and psychiatry is the Bliss Classification, mentioned above. It is used in a number of Australian and British libraries, but so far it has had almost no influence on bibliographic organization in general (Editorial, 1960).

The third problem poses the question whether psychology can be confined within the traditional classification of the sciences or whether it calls for another organizing principle to supplement this classification. In 1906, Carl Stumpf, professor of psychology in Berlin, acknowledged the dilemma by observing that, for the whole modern systematization of science, psychology proved to be a somewhat inconvenient subject. During the greater part of this century, which witnessed the most spectacular growth of psychology, the problem did not come nearer to a solution. B. M. Kedrov (1956), a Russian authority on the history and philosophy of science, noted that psychology could not be completely assigned to the social, nor to the natural, nor to the philosophical sciences, although being closely linked to each of them. This author concluded that psychology had, after all, the closest links with philosophy. A similar position has more recently been stated in India by S. R. Ranganathan, author of the Colon Classification which is internationally respected because of its novel approach to the many-faceted nature of books. He reaffirmed that psychology, while a borderline case and belonging in part to the social sciences, must be assigned to the humanities in view of its genesis in philosophy (Seetharama, 1965). Although the seventeenth edition of the Dewey Decimal Classification of 1965 contains a completely new schedule for psychology, psychology was again left in the class "Philosophy and Related Disciplines." This international consensus cannot be ignored.

At one time most sciences had their origin in philosophy which, even in the 20th century, has repeatedly supported the movement for the unity of science. The relations between modern physics and philosophy are also close, but this is not construed as a reason for subordinating physics to philosophy. To recognize the bonds between philosophy and psychology alone means isolating psychology from both the biomedical and the social sciences and, in many instances, from the humanities as well. As a result, assigning psychology to philosophy takes it out of the context of recent intellectual history which has given the psychological sciences a vital role in the striving for unity of the behavioral sciences. The practical implications go far beyond the physical dispersion of the books. A library's classification system governs not only its catalogs but also many other operations such as acquisition policies, the practice of selecting books, and statistics of their use. Since the old historical framework cannot reflect the contemporary scientific relationships, a different bibliographic system is needed to complement the present classification of psychology and to counteract its unwanted effects.

## FROM THE PSYCHOLOGICAL TO THE BEHAVIORAL SCIENCES

In the broadest sense, the behavioral sciences aim at developing a general theory of human behavior on the basis of facts gathered by a variety of scientific approaches (Miller, 1955). When the new term is applied in the most limited sense, the behavioral sciences are equated with one part of the social sciences, including only sociology, anthropology, and social psychology. Between these two extremes there are varied interpretations of the phrase "behavioral sciences" (Senn, 1966). The specific meaning can often be ascertained only from the context, but in some form the psychological sciences are always represented. It has been suggested that the behavioral sciences be defined as

> a multidisciplinary pursuit of knowledge about behavior in its roots and manifestations, in man and animals, in individuals, groups, and cultures, and in all conditions, normal, exceptional, and pathological (Editorial, 1960, p. 701).

In terms of a unifying theory, these are all aspects of behavior but in practice the specific subjects are studied within one or another of the established sectors of science.

A bibliographic system to be developed for the behavioral science literature should be able to show its multiple relevance: publications which contribute to the behavioral sciences as a comprehensive area of study are, at the same time, works on a particular subject; they embody the approaches of a variety of disciplines but may have to use the disciplinary channels of scientific literature and communication. For purposes of behavioral science bibliography, the subject approach to books as now used in libraries is neither superfluous nor sufficient.

## AN ORBITAL SYSTEM AS BIBLIOGRAPHIC-ORGANIZING PRINCIPLE

An organizing principle for the behavioral science literature should be based on the following premises: The behavioral sciences are concerned with man as a whole; they study the behavior of man and of animals and may search for knowledge about man in relation to any conditions in the world around him, those prior to his existence and those created or modified by him; they are characterized by a mode of scientific inquiry that involves the interaction of other fields with the psychological sciences: psychology, psychiatry, and psychoanalysis.

This mode of inquiry may serve as a criterion for distinguishing the behavioral science literature from the general literature of the sciences of man which include all biomedical and social sciences, philosophy, religion, and many other fields. The interaction occurs in various forms and degrees, for example: (a) when a fusion between the psychological sciences and other disciplines creates a new, independent field such as neurochemistry or psycholinguistics; (b) when the psychological sciences draw on knowledge obtained by nonpsychological methods; (c) when other fields use the concepts, methods, or theories of the psychological sciences; and (d) when other fields absorb the pertinent findings of the psychological sciences, while retaining their own general structure and function, as, for instance, education.

Accordingly, the new organizing principle should be orbital, not linear. It should place the psychological sciences in the center of the system that is being organized, thereby integrating the anthropocentric and the anthropotropic approaches. It should allow other fields to find their place in an orbital position, depending on the degree of interaction with the psychological sciences. The system should be open, allowing for relationships that may develop with fields beyond the biological and social sciences and with fields that may be added to the present spectrum of the sciences through future discoveries.

Such an orbital bibliographic organization would make it possible to identify and trace the various bodies of literature which develop within the behavioral sciences as here defined. The system would unify and make evident the body of knowledge produced by the psychological sciences and their fusion with other fields. This would provide a focus for observing the progress of basic knowledge about human behavior. It would also show the growing scope of knowledge that becomes relevant to the psychological sciences, but it would select only the pertinent material from the literature of disciplines which pursue scientific goals of their own. By tracing the applications of the new knowledge to other fields, the growing influence of the behavioral sciences could be observed. The orbital system would thus delineate the network of cross-classifications which scientists expect from modern documentation and which is considered one of its most urgent needs. If the various bodies of literature were so identified and viewed together, the progress of inquiry achieved by the behavioral sciences and its impact would become apparent.

It is important for scientific and practical reasons to organize the behavioral science literature in a way that permits keeping the necessary distinctions clear. To equate this literature with the total literature of some or all fields concerned with man would dilute and destroy the meaning of the new scientific conception. The first requirement is, therefore, to delimit the behavioral science literature in general in a functional sense. It is no less important to recognize, in each area of specialization, the works which are linked to the behavioral sciences. In fields where the need to understand human behavior is practical and direct, such as, particularly, the health sciences, law, religion, education, business, and politics, there is a growing number of works which present their material in the light of the findings of the behavioral sciences. Since the subject approach now used in libraries and general bibliographies does not single out such publications, they need to be identified through additional bibliographic techniques and guides.

When the evolving behavioral science literature is so delimited and differentiated, its bibliography could serve the relevant purposes of the scientific community, national and international planning of research, educational planning and curriculum design, presentation of significant developments to the nonspecialists and the general public, and contemporary library organization.

Planning for a new bibliographic system must take into account the existence of computers which could combine the data obtained through such different approaches as the classified and the orbital form of bibliographic organization. It is urgent to consider these possibilities before the programming of computers proceeds too far within the existing limited framework. The corrective devices now available to librarians cannot be applied when computers accept and freeze every anachronism in the bibliographic data they process. Computer programs in bibliography must be attuned to the fundamentals of a science and must stay abreast of changes in theory and concepts. This requirement is now widely recognized in principle. The problems encountered in organizing the literature of the behavioral sciences will also throw some light upon this larger issue.

In a pilot study, a new system for the monographic literature of the behavioral sciences has been developed over the past 10 years by the *Mental Health Book Review Index*. The journals indexed for reviews relate more or less closely to the behavioral sciences. The groups of reviews cited include at least one evaluation from a journal in the psychological sciences and reflect the collective judgments of the scientific community, which indicate the degrees of relevance to the central concepts of the behavioral sciences.

The orbital organization of the emerging behavioral science literature, if carried out on a larger scale, could lead to the bibliographic reorientation which is proposed here. It would take the form of a superstructure that complements, but does not attempt to replace the basic bibliographic and library organization. It would no longer deny the existence of dilemmas nor accept defeat. By using a pluralistic approach rather than trying to enforce a single structure, it would provide an open system and allow new contributions to fall into place.

## REFERENCES

American Psychological Association. Proceedings of the 39th annual meeting, Toronto, Ontario, September 10, 11, 12, 1931. *Psychological Bulletin,* 1931, **28,** 649-712.

Bliss, H. E. *A bibliographic classification.* New York: Wilson, 1952-53. 4 vols.

Coulson, T. An outline of the theory of classification. *Library World,* 1911, **14,** 37-42, 67-70.

Delay, J. *Aspects de la psychiatrie moderne.* Paris: Presses universitaires de France, 1956.

Dubuc, R. Les "sciences de l'homme" dans la CDU. *Revue Internationale de la Documentation,* 1963, **30,** 137-140.

Editorial. The behavioral sciences and mental health in relation to the organization of knowledge, the organization of science, and bibliography. *AMA Archives of General Psychiatry,* 1960, **2,** 701-706. (Reprinted from *Mental Health Book Review Index,* 1960, **5**(1), i-v.)

Grinker, R. R. *Psychosomatic research.* New York: Norton, 1953.

Grolier, E. de. L'Etude des problèmes de classification documentaire sur le plan international. *Review of Documentation,* 1953, **20,** 105-117.

Kedrov, B. La classification des sciences. *Recherches Soviétiques,* 1956, No. 1, 83-111.

MacKenzie, R. C., and Bloomquist, H. The impact of the behavioral sciences on the collecting policy of medical school libraries. Appendix: Master list of journals relating to the behavioral sciences in the Harvard Medical Library. *Bulletin of the Medical Library Association,* 1964, **52,** 220-233.

Miller, J. G. Toward a general theory for the behavioral sciences. *American Psychologist,* 1955, **10,** 513-531.

Petzholdt, J. Bibliographische Systeme. In his *Bibliotheca bibliographica.* Leipzig: W. Engelmann, 1866, Pp. 20-65.

Seetharama, R. Social sciences in Colon classification. *Herald of Library Science,* 1965, **4,** 91-96.

Senn, P. R. What is "behavioral science?"—Notes toward a history. *J. of the History of the Behavioral Sciences,* 1966, **2,** 107-122.

Warren. H. C. Memorandum anent revised Dewey classification. *Psychological Bulletin,* 1931, **28,** 198.

# ESSAY 9

## *Links Between the Humanities and the Literature of the Human Sciences*

Originally published as Editorial in *Mental Health Book Review Index,* vol. 11 (whole no. 16), 1966. Reprinted here in an expanded version and with a bibliography by permission from the January 1968 issue of the *Wilson Library Bulletin.* 

The humanities in the modern sense, as man's accomplishments in literature and art, philosophy and religion, are thousands of years older than the human sciences, which have emerged during the past hundred years as the scientific study of man himself. In Western Civilization, the humanities in another sense, as the study of the Greek and Roman classics, had earlier been pursued under different names, but the term "humanities" had its origin in the Renaissance. In the process of secularization that followed the Middle Ages, "humanity" as a field of learning was set off from "divinity." In our time, the concern with the scientific study of man arises from a background of three centuries of modern science. The contrast now is between the physical sciences, which view man as a part of nature, and the human sciences, which view him "as a person."[1]

The new term "human sciences," along with the related "behavioral sciences," came into use during the 1950's. Both terms signify an endeavor to unify the evolving knowledge centered on man and imply that man has added to his study of nature and his mastery of machines the study and intended mastery of his own behavior.[2] This point has been graphically made by Bernard Berelson and Gary A. Steiner, who, in their *Human Behavior,* have tried to identify the new scientific findings. Noting that the twentieth century marks the coming-of-age of the behavioral sciences, the authors suggest "that the more intimate (to man) the subject matter, the younger the science. Astronomy before geography, physical science before biology, medicine before psychology—even though in each case the availability of data was in the reverse order."[3]

## HUMANISTIC UNDERCURRENTS

This essay illustrates a trend in that part of the current nonfiction literature which, though primarily concerned with the study of human behavior, is also related in some way to the humanities in the contemporary sense.[4] Thousands of works in the psychological sciences dealing directly with literature and art have already been recorded.[5] The scope of scholarly work relevant to the human sciences and the humanities is, however, broader than that; it involves a greater variety of scientific approaches and the study of many other humanistic topics. Scholars in the human sciences also turn sometimes to the humanities in the course of work that is clearly a subject of psychological and social research. There is at present no direct bibliographic approach to a study of the humanistic aspects in the literature of the human sciences.[6] The extent and direction of this trend can only be inferred from examining books selected for this purpose. This is the approach we have used here.

Our working sample comes from a continuous annual bibliography of books and book reviews in the behavioral sciences, the *Mental Health Book Review Index.*[7] The *Index* is a cooperative project, in which nearly fifty librarians in this country and Canada participate. It presents a bibliographic record of books that have aroused sufficient interest to result in a substantial, cross-disciplinary evaluation in the book review literature of the behavioral sciences. Each annual volume of the *Index* lists some three hundred such books with references to all their reviews found in two hundred journals in the English language. Books become eligible for listing in the *Index* when there are three or more authoritative reviews from journals representing various psychological and other disciplines.

This essay is based on the eleventh volume of the *Mental Health Book Review Index* (1966). From this cross section of works selected and evaluated by the specialists who assess the literature of the behavioral sciences as a whole, we chose those books in which some relation to the humanities could be found. Therefore, the weight which our examples carry can be judged by considering the place these books hold in the current literature of the human sciences.

The present article groups and reviews these examples and considers some of the issues involved in each group. The main issue, however, is the implicit challenge to find ways of identifying the emergent humanistically oriented literature which the examples illustrate and outline. This literature is not defined by subject, discipline, or field of knowledge. It derives its identity and unity from giving expression to the "quest for the rediscovery of man,"[8] that makes it relevant to the human sciences and to the humanities.

## CREATIVE WRITERS AND HUMAN SCIENTISTS

In 1907, when Freud published the first psychoanalytic study of a novel, Wilhelm Jensen's *Gradiva,* he sounded a basic theme: "creative writers are valuable allies and their evidence is to be prized highly. . . . In their knowledge of the mind they are far in advance of us everyday people, for they draw upon sources which we have not yet opened up for science."[9] Almost sixty years later, Sir Cyril Burt virtually seconds Freud's appraisal. In his foreword to Arthur Koestler's *The Act of Creation,* he warns the student of human nature not to forget "that most of what we know about the mind of man is to be learnt from the writings not of scientists but of men of letters—the poets and the philosophers, the biographers and the historians, the novelists and the literary critics."[10]

The human sciences have transformed contemporary literature, changed the interpretation of older literary and religious documents, and used the humanities as a resource for insights into psychological and social problems. Social scientists have invaded a domain long claimed by the "humanists" by studying the relationships between people, as noted in a book of readings and essays entitled *Interpersonal Dynamics.* The editors, Warren G. Bennis and others, have made their selections with an eye to the teacher and student of interpersonal relations as well as to the intelligent layman. They hope these relationships can be improved when they are better understood. In his foreword to this volume, Douglas McGregor commends the editors "for transcending (some will say violating) the existing norms concerning the distinctions between science and the humanities." They have chosen, for example, the "perceptive and fascinating tale" by George Orwell, "Shooting the Elephant," to illustrate the "oft-quoted wisdom that 'people become what you expect them to be.' " The inclusion of fiction in such a reader also illustrates McGregor's point that the slow process of accumulating useful knowledge about man's behavior is well served by the observations of behavior reflected in the work of a first-class novelist and by those reflected in the report of a scientific research study.[11]

The authors of current works in the human sciences make use of fiction and poetry in various other ways. Sylvia Brody adds "Footnotes from Literature" to her psychoanalytic study of passivity in boys. There she brings together passages from Keats, Poe, and other poets and writers, which have in common a theme that expresses the wish for passive surrender.[12] J. H. van den Berg considers that the European literature as a whole supports his theory about "historical psychology," which he presents in *The Changing Nature of Man.* He has drawn upon literary sources of different periods to show that man changes and that psychology must adopt a historical perspective on human nature. He regards maturation, for example, "as evidence of the distance between young and old" and claims that, before Rousseau, this subject was almost totally absent from all European literature because maturation was then "an absent phase of life." Berg suggests that the German word *Flegeljahre* ("boorish years," used by Jean Paul as the title of a novel) and even the very phenomenon of psychological symptoms of puberty and of adolescence was new around 1800. His explanation also puts in perspective Victor Hugo's remark: "Columbus only discovered America; it was I who discovered the child."[13]

Other authors make critical comments on literature from their point of view as social scientists. For example, in *A Reader for Parents,* prepared under the auspices of the Child Study Association of America, Anna W. M. Wolf traces the major phases of childhood through selections from Proust, Faulkner, James Joyce, Colette, and other creative writers. She notes in her introduction that Freudian insights, which pervade the literature of today, are "often so perfectly wedded to the genius of the artist that we are scarcely aware of the union," and contends that we have accepted these insights so fully "that we even tend to judge the psychologic vision of earlier writers by the extent to which they anticipate Freud."[14]

## PSYCHOLOGICAL STUDY OF PERSONAL DOCUMENTS

In his book *Stigma,* in which personal accounts describing the experience of social rejection are gleaned from various sources, the sociologist Erving Goffman also draws upon fiction. He criticizes some fictionalized presentations of such an experience as being candid to the point of exposure and betrayal because the most deeply hidden sores of the stigmatized "are touched on and examined in the clinical manner that is a current literary fashion." Goffman names James Baldwin as an example in regard to Negroes, and Hector Chevigny, in regard to the blind.[15] Most of those who consider fiction as relevant to psychological research look for basic similarities. However, Margaret Phillips, a British social scientist who has studied small groups, finds a basic difference between pertinent novels and her own work. She points out that novelists such as Sir Hugh Walpole, Nigel Balchin, and Sir Charles Snow, who have taken small groups as their subject, see the group as a network of interacting individuals, while she sees the group as itself an entity that can be observed in conditions of adversity and other real life situations.[16]

Another type of study applies psychological knowledge to autobiographical writings. *The Universal Experience of Adolescence* by Norman Kiell is organized in chapters that reflect certain characteristics of adolescent development such as the adolescent's tendency to contradictions and his need to conform to his peers. The author traces these patterns through more than two hundred autobiographies, diaries, and letters, ranging from Marcus Aurelius to Graham Greene, from Marie Bashkirtseff to Anne Frank, to show that this development "is basically uniform in all societies." A bibliography of more than a thousand items, "Psychology, Psychoanalysis and Personal Documents," extends the book's scope beyond its special theme.[17]

Carney Landis devoted many years to a diligent search for autobiographical accounts of the experience of those who have lived through a period of insanity. Assisted by a German and a French psychologist, he had finally located and read some two hundred books and an equal number of journal articles that were such first-hand accounts. No comprehensive collection of such writings had previously appeared in print. In 1964, however, when his book *Varieties of Psychopathological Experience*[18] was posthumously published, another American psychologist, Bert Kaplan, published *The Inner World of Mental Illness,* "a series of first-person accounts of what it was like."[19] Although there is considerable overlap in the sources used by the two authors, the books differ so greatly that they supplement rather than duplicate each other. Landis chose to organize and discuss his material in the fashion of a textbook. His excerpts are brief and scattered through separate chapters, even when they come from the same source, to illustrate the various forms of mental illness, a presentation which is further highlighted by a "diagnostic index." Kaplan introduces only briefly his lengthy excerpts, each of which leaves the unity of the original document intact. His collection includes excerpts from works by Saint Augustine, Feodor Dostoevsky, Leo Tolstoi, and Jean-Paul Sartre, which shed light upon such experiences as depersonalization and depression. (These writers are also represented in selections made by other authors who offer a different psychological focus: on childhood, on adolescence, and on the personalities of eminent men.[20]

While both Landis and Kaplan present and explore the body of psychopathological literature, several of the works they cite have long been individually known. Clifford Beers' *A Mind That Found Itself,* in particular, has become a classic that is still widely read. In a letter that first appeared in the original edition of 1908, William James wrote, "It reads like fiction, but it is not fiction." Beers used the experience of his own insanity and recovery to set in motion the mental hygiene movement, through which he attained a position of international leadership.[21] *The Locomotive-God,* written in the 1920's by William Ellery Leonard, an American poet and professor of English literature, is also internationally known as a classic account of a lifelong phobia, which the author traced to a terrifying episode in his childhood.[22]

New accounts of personal encounters with mental illness continue to appear. *Beyond All Reason* is an autobiographical document, written under the pseudonym Morag Coate, by a schizophrenic patient who "became mad five times in fourteen years." The British psychiatrist R. D. Laing, himself an author of books in the area of existentialism and psychiatry, has written a deeply sympathetic foreword. He stresses the need for a book such as this that gives a picture of what it is to be a schizophrenic person rather than a schizophrenic case. Therefore, he considers it as useful to those who come in contact with such patients through family and community care and in mental hospitals. Since the book raises issues "within a domain of relevance that takes us to the very horizons of human existence," Laing thinks it has relevance also to theologians, priests, and philosophers.[23] Another development within this literature is suggested in the book *And Always Tomorrow* by Sarah E. Lorenz, which is also a pseudonym. Here the mother of a boy who became mentally ill at the age of sixteen gives an account of seven years of a most dedicated search for a cure. The parents, willing to subject their son "to every conceivable form of therapy," at one time even completely involve themselves by participating in the family research program conducted in a national institution.[24] Besides such autobiographical accounts, there are psychiatric studies of a personal document written by an insane person. A notable example of a work containing both the document and its interpretation is Macalpine and Hunter's book *Schizophrenia 1677*, discussed in some detail later.[25]

Biography written from the medical or psychiatric point of view flourished in the latter part of the nineteenth century. This literature became so extensive, especially in Europe, that the term *Pathographie* was coined in Germany for these publications, many of which tried to establish relationships between genius and mental illness. To a large extent, the approach has changed in the twentieth century and has led to a new genre, "psychobiography." Two recent examples of the psychoanalytic scrutiny of autobiographies, memoirs, letters, diaries, and other records of famous persons in the arts and sciences are Kurt Eissler's *Goethe*[26] and the study of Darwin and Samuel Butler made by Phyllis Greenacre "as a contribution to the understanding of the creative individual."[27]

Biographical data about men of letters play a role in psychological studies in various other contexts. In his book *Spatial Ability*, Ian Macfarlane Smith deals with the significance and measurement of spatial, as opposed to verbal, ability and appends to his text personal data about men whose special achievement is known. He points out how spatial and verbal abilities correspond to certain personality traits which vary for such groups as writers, artists, and scientists. In noting these personality differences, he suggests in passing that the phenomenon of the "two cultures"–the concept regarding the gulf between scientists and nonscientists introduced by C. P. Snow in his now famous Rede Lecture of 1959–is not peculiar to our own generation. As a personalized illustration of the mutual antipathy between a humanist and a scientist, he recalls that Sydney Smith described Sir Humphrey Davy as a "very foolish coxcomb out of his crucibles," while the chemist Davy dubbed the English essayist and preacher "an affable jester concealed under the gown of the sacred minister of religion."[28] On the basis of his study of one thousand eminent men, I. D. Harris proposes that firstborn sons characteristically differ from later sons in personality makeup and outlook. He also tries to show that his hypothesis applies to first and later sons eminent in literature, history, or science, for each area in a specific way.[29] For their book *Cradles of Eminence,* Victor and Mildred Goertzel, using biographies, studied the childhood of four hundred famous persons living in the twentieth century. About half of these persons contributed in some way to the humanities. The authors report as one of their findings that 90 of 105 writers of fiction, drama, or poetry saw, as children, tense psychological dramas played out by their parents.[30] Studies of this kind, which ascertain historical and biographical facts in the course of psychological or social research, produce new bodies of data pertaining to the humanities.

## FANTASY AND CREATIVITY AS TOPICS OF RESEARCH

The human sciences have also turned to various subjects that formerly were the sole province of the humanities. Fantasy is one such subject. Heuscher's *A Psychiatric Study of Fairy Tales* is largely concerned with an application of psychoanalytic concepts. In addition, it touches on cultural trends, noting, for example, that more than 350 variants of the "Cinderella" story exist in various parts of the world. One chapter relates fairy tales to westerns, crime stories, and television.[31] In their *Children Tell Stories,* Evelyn G. Pitcher and Ernst Prelinger analyze the fantasy of nursery and kindergarten children not in relation to the stories they absorb by listening, reading, or watching the screen, but to those they tell. Margaret Lowenfeld suggests in her foreword to this book that some of these stories may come from the deeper level that gives rise to fairy tales of universal appeal and cites "the story from a four-year-old girl, which seems to express the association of feminine sexuality and the sea which appears so often in myths." In a final comment, the authors show concern that their "analyses and interpretations have fallen short of doing justice to or even of comprehending the complexity, the richness, and the literary quality, poetry, and beauty which many of the stories contain."[32]

The nature of creativity also has fascinated many scholars in the humanities and in the human sciences. The concept of creativity is still changing. Arthur Koestler, in his treatise *The Act of Creation,* finds a basic pattern in all human creative activities, in art, science, and literature, and looks for basic principles that are at work in creative activities on all levels of organic life.[33] In current psychological research, human creativity has been studied in relation to other human capacities, for example, intelligence. Formerly, literary and art criticism considered only the artistic qualities of a work. The scope of this criticism was later extended to explore psychological or psychoanalytic implications.[34] More recently, the psychological sciences have added a concern with the qualities of character and personality that are often needed to bring a great work to fruition. In his book *Creativity and Psychological Health,* Frank Barron points to what he calls simply, " 'the moral attitude.' " He suggests that creative writers have a profound commitment to larger aesthetic and philosophical meanings and that "without this intense cosmological commitment no amount of mental ability of the sort measured by I.Q. tests will suffice to produce a genuinely creative act."[35] In *Guiding Creative Talent,* E. Paul Torrance, who is particularly concerned with the challenge creativity poses to education, draws on imaginative stories of school children to illustrate personality patterns often found in children with creative talent. For example, he detects an ability to cope with failure and frustration in the persistence that marks the story written by a fifth-grade Negro boy from Georgia: A monkey was very sad because he didn't know how to fly, while other animals did. He climbed up a tree, jumped out, and fell to the ground. He did it again, and again, and finally he began to fly. Torrance comments: "Certainly, almost all highly creative scientists, inventors, artists, and writers attempt tasks which are too difficult for them. Had they not attempted such tasks, it is quite unlikely that their great ideas would have been born."[36]

Creativity extends beyond the verbal sphere. Like children's stories, children's drawings have been collected with a view to studying their universal significance. D. B. Harris includes a historical review of such international research undertakings carried out prior to World War I, and of other pertinent psychological studies, in his book *Children's Drawings as Measures of Intellectual Maturity.*[37] The fine arts and music, though latecomers to scholarship in the humanities, have long been praised for their healing capacity and expressive power, qualities that have gained them a special place in the human sciences. To the psychological study of works of art[38] and music, there has been added the use of art and music as a form of therapy. The illustrated *Bulletin of Art Therapy* and the *Journal of Music Therapy* may serve as current sources for articles and bibliographies. As reminders of this great faculty that music has, "to console, to comfort . . . to take us out of ourselves," Joseph Szigeti recalls, in a paper contributed to the symposium *Conflict and Creativity,* the almost identical titles of two books in his library, *Trösterin Musica* (an expression of Martin Luther's) and *La Musique Consolatrice* by Georges Duhamel.[39]

The study of paintings and drawings of the mentally ill has become another field of specialization in the psychological sciences. *Schizophrenia 1677* has already been mentioned as an autobiographical account subjected to psychiatric interpretation. In 1677, the painter Christoph Haizmann eloquently illustrated the story of his encounter with the Devil. Freud had access to the unpublished manuscript and analyzed the psychosis. Now that the original text has been published by Ida Macalpine and R. A. Hunter, with color reproductions of the nine remarkable paintings that depict the development of the patient's illness, the document has become available to historically oriented psychiatrists and to those who may wish "to observe Freud working on a case history and . . . to argue the case with Freud."[40]

Many of these topics, particularly children's literature, drawings, paintings, and music—American, Balinese, Chinese, French, German—enter into the comparative study of culture. In their collection of such studies, *Childhood in Contemporary Cultures,* Margaret Mead and Martha Wolfenstein devote one section to "Fantasies for and about Children"[41] and explore also "the ways in which children are depicted in current films of different countries."[42]

## COMMUNICATION RESEARCH

Research in the area of communication appears to be shifting from the humanities to the human sciences, though this trend is not easy to follow. Studies of language, humor, and other modes of communication often continue to be considered as part of the humanities when the emphasis is on normal behavior and development. They are thus separated from works concerned with communication that is disturbed or takes place in a clinical setting. The slow pace of unifying knowledge about man, "in all conditions, normal, exceptional, and pathological,"[43] seems to be even slower when this knowledge reaches man's need to express himself and to communicate with others.

The following examples of books that would now be claimed by the communication sciences suggest the broadening range of this field. Language remains the subject of central interest. Psychologists in the field of child development present their studies of language and symbol formation in relation to the development of thought.[44] Other authors deal with aphasia[45] and related disturbances of language, speech, and the ability to read. The British neurologist Macdonald Critchley, who was chairman of an international symposium on *Disorders of Language,*[46] also wrote a monograph on *Developmental Dyslexia,*[47] a concept that has replaced that of "congenital word-blindness." From the point of view of educators who are also psychologists, Florence Roswell and Gladys Natchez deal with this subject in *Reading Disability*[48] (the broader and now popular term). The authors of both these books succeed in putting vividly before the reader the human and humanistic aspects of this condition. The two books supplement each other, sometimes even on specific points. For example, Roswell and Natchez present the case history of a twelve-year-old boy who has difficulties with spelling as well as reading. He begins to improve when he reads about Hans Christian Andersen's anxieties and feelings of rejection, and takes hope for himself when he learns that "The Ugly Duckling" is a story about Andersen's own life. Critchley mentions the belief that Andersen was himself a dyslexic and illustrates it with a table of his characteristic spelling errors.

There are new ways of studying communication as a form of human behavior and human relations. For example, William F. Fry's *Sweet Madness: a Study of Humor* does not deal with humor as part of literature, but attempts to arrive at a theory of humor. The author, a psychiatrist, has based his book on research he had earlier conducted within a program of communication research at the Department of Anthropology at Stanford University.[49] The authors of *The Therapeutic Dialogue,* Jerome L. Schulman and others, present a new method for analyzing the verbal interaction between therapist and patient, an approach that relates psychotherapy to research in communication.[50]

Sometimes the developments under study are new themselves. In *The People Look at Educational Television,* Wilbur Schramm and others report the results of analyzing more than thirty thousand interviews, a contribution from the Institute for Communication Research at Stanford University.[51] C. A. Thomas and his coauthors, however, who in their *Programmed Learning in Perspective* offer a guide to program writing as another recent branch of communication science, also take us back to some older fundamentals. For example, they see programmed learning as an individual learning process that incorporates in revised form Socratic and Cartesian methods.[52]

Through research in communication, the humanities are now linked not only with education and rehabilitation, psychology, psychiatry, and neurology, as here suggested, but also with other fields in the social and biological sciences. A number of journals reflect these broadening relationships. The *Journal of Communication,* for example, now regularly provides an annotated bibliography on the multidisciplinary "Current Developments in Communication Research," and the *American Anthropologist* includes "Linguistics" in its classified book review section.[53]

## TRENDS IN PHILOSOPHY AND RELIGION

Philosophy and religion, claimed by the humanities in the broadest sense, have stimulated the human sciences and have been modernized in contact with them. Henri Baruk relates the ancient documents of Hebraic civilization to the contemporary science of man,[54] while Hans Jacobs confronts Freud and Jung with Hindu philosophy.[55] Three journals reflect the impact of existentialism: *Existential Psychiatry, Journal of Existentialism,* and *Review of Existential Psychology and Psychiatry.* Joseph Lyons refers to his *Psychology and the Measure of Man* as "a book that touches on phenomenology and existentialism," and to psychology as a "humanistic science." This book aims at a clinical science of man; it is written, however, with "a poeticizing orientation" and begins with an essay on the poet and his reader, in which Lyons contrasts the textbook approach with "the overriding experience we sometimes achieve when we share with a poet his grasp of some truth."[56]

An international trend is particularly apparent in this converging of psychological and philosophical schools of thought. Caruso's *Existential Psychology* was translated from the German,[57] Strasser's *Phenomenology and the Human Sciences,* from the Dutch.[58] Books in the series "Studies in Existential Analysis and Phenomenology," which originate in England, have also appeared in this country.[59] Besides forming part of the Rice University Semicentennial Celebration in 1962, the symposium on *Behaviorism and Phenomenology,* edited by T. W. Wann, was chosen to mark the inception of the new Division of Philosophical Psychology in the American Psychological Association.[60]

The study of religion in the light of the psychological sciences has become a special field. Books in this field reflect two major trends—a marked rise of academic research pertaining to religion, and an endeavor to cultivate the area of human problems that is of common concern to the clergy and professional groups engaged in psychotherapy. Both trends have flourished periodically since the latter part of the nineteenth century, although neither with the impetus nor with the impact attained during the 1960's.[61]

As the following examples suggest, the underlying trends, while still distinct, often overlap, and the problems that come to light in the borderland between religion and the human sciences are apt to be delicate and subtle. Religion and death are two of nine subjects covered in the book *Taboo Topics,* edited by Norman L. Farberow.[62] Although social scientists have been reluctant to enter into certain realms of inner experience, the recurrent resistance to studying human behavior in relation to religion and in the confrontation with death is again being overcome. This is shown, for example, by Margaretta K. Bowers in *Conflicts of the Clergy,* a study with case histories based on her experience as a psychotherapist, and in *Counseling the Dying,* a book in which she combines her own insights, gained by her experience as a practicing physician, with those of three coauthors who contribute theological, pastoral, psychological, and other relevant perspectives.[63]

In historical perspective, William Douglas has analyzed the complex difficulties surrounding the study of "the religious quest as a valid aspect of human behavior." He makes a point similar to that of Berelson and Steiner,[64] whom we quoted earlier: that the study of what he calls the " 'out-there' " precedes that of the " 'in-here.' " Special difficulties arise for the researcher who, instead of investigating the religion of distant cultures and historical periods, studies the normal religious experience in his own cultural setting. Douglas also finds that interest in the scientific study of religion, while strong in the first quarter of the twentieth century and again since 1950, was not encouraged within the social sciences during the interval 1925 to 1950. He suggests that the objections then raised against the study of religion applied also to the work of all those concerned with the " 'humanistic'—as distinguished from the strictly experimental and/or 'valueless,' descriptive—approach to social science."[65]

Michael Argyle has covered the same period in *Religious Behavior,* "a study in the social psychology of religion in Britain and America since 1900." He has made a synthesis of data from many statistical sources to show how religious behavior and belief vary with such factors as personality traits and attitudes, influences of the environment, age, sex, and social class, and he uses these findings to test psychoanalytic and other theories of religion.[66] The literature of the religio-psychiatric movement, which "concerns the relation between religious and psychological ideas about emotional disturbances," forms the basis for Samuel Z. Klausner's book *Psychiatry and Religion.* This is a detailed, largely statistical study of writings of ministers and psychiatrists "bridging the fields of religion and of psychiatry in their concern with mental or spiritual health." One of Klausner's tables shows that, in the decade from 1948 to 1957, a total of 851 books and articles in religion and psychiatry were published, as compared to 65 in the decade from 1918 to 1927.[67] Together, these three historical studies suggest that, around 1960, a growing number of scholars in the psychological and social sciences were so deeply concerned with religion that some of them began to take stock by tracing the long-term trend since the beginning of the twentieth century.

In a different way, two works dealing with primitive forms of the priest-doctor role and related religious behavior throughout the world supplement each other. Mircea Eliade uses the approach of a historian of religion in his comprehensive work *Shamanism: Archaic Techniques of Ecstasy.* He suggests that a knowledge of this whole spiritual world that differs from our own "is a necessity for every true humanist," adding that humanism has for some time ceased to be identified only with the spiritual tradition of the West.[68] Cultural anthropologists and social psychiatrists share an interest in the study of religious beliefs and rituals, as found now in primitive cultures and underdeveloped societies, when these beliefs have a bearing on psychological treatment. Ari Kiev has edited an anthology of such contemporary studies entitled *Magic, Faith, and Healing.*[69]

Psychological approaches to religion as an intimate human experience are apt to span a wider range than other studies of human behavior. Abraham H. Maslow, currently president of the American Psychological Association, presents his Kappa Delta Pi Lecture, *Religions, Values, and Peak-Experiences,* somewhat as a "progress report" in the course of his "investigations of psychological health for the theory of values, of ethics, of education, of psychotherapy, of 'religion,' of work, etc." He defines peak-experiences as "secularized religious or mystical or transcendent experiences," which can be investigated by psychologists. What mystical or peak-experiences and all religions have in common in their essence, Maslow calls the "core-religious experience" or the "transcendent experience." It is one of his conclusions that the teaching of spiritual and ethical values has a place in education and in other social institutions.[70] In contrast, religion as an element in paranoid delusion enters into a research project in social psychology and personality theory, conducted by Milton Rokeach. He describes in *The Three Christs of Ypsilanti*[71] his study in which three schizophrenic patients in a Michigan State Hospital, each claiming to be Christ, were brought together for two years in daily confrontation.

Like the series "Religious Perspectives,"[72] much of the new scholarly concern with religion "represents a quest for the rediscovery of man."[73] Eliade spells this out, as he reminds the historian of religion that "the phenomena with which he is concerned reveal boundary-line situations of mankind, and that these situations demand to be understood and made understandable."[74] This fundamental issue emerges also from the controversy concerning the right to, and the dangers of, mystical experience allegedly brought about by so-called "consciousness-expanding" or other drugs. Four recent books on LSD have put this question before a larger public.[75] Since the theme of such experience has its own tradition in literature, it is hardly surprising that two of the four books, *The Psychedelic Experience* by Timothy Leary and others, and the collection of articles on *LSD: the Consciousness-Expanding Drug,* edited by David Solomon, are dedicated to Aldous Huxley, the best-known creative writer on drugs and their psychological effects in our time.[76]

As we have shown, creative writers, artists, humanistic scholars, and human scientists freely cross into one another's domain. Their relationships need not and often cannot be interdisciplinary in the formal sense. If the links that are being formed escape attention, this may be due to a conventional way of looking at the arts and sciences, which separates that which might be joined. Attempts to add an element of art to the literature of the human sciences have been most elusive, although they express perhaps most strongly the longing to humanize, not science itself, but rather the impact of science upon mankind.

## POETIC OVERTONES

It has been common practice for novelists and playwrights to choose a poetic—sometimes a biblical—quotation for a title. Only recently, however, have writers in the human sciences begun to use a poetic phrase for the title before revealing, in the subtitle, the actual content of the book. The titles of the following five books, for example, were drawn from English poetry: *So Fair a House* (Casriel: "The Story of Synanon")[77] and *Unwillingly to School* (Kahn and Nursten: "The Place of the Child Guidance Clinic in the Treatment of School Phobia")[78] are the words of Shakespeare, while *Sweet Madness* (Fry: "A Study of Humor")[79] and *The Promised Seed* (Harris: "A Comparative Study of Eminent First and Later Sons")[80] come from Milton. For *This Island Now,* his B.B.C. Reith Lectures of 1962 that probed into social changes in the twentieth century,[81] G. M. Carstairs took a theme from a poem by W. H. Auden of the 1930's (first included in Auden's *Look Stranger!* and *On This Island*) and echoed the line: "Look, stranger, on this island now."[82] Through allusions to poetry, Carstairs tried to express his sense of "the importance of keeping intellectually abreast with events in a fast-changing world community, while still keeping imaginatively in touch with the creative artists. . . ." In listening to these overtones, may we conclude that, as we enter the last third of the twentieth century, the human sciences are coming of age and are now free to acknowledge their forerunners, their ancestors, and their masters in the humanities?

## NOTES

1. Stephen Strasser. *Phenomenology and the Human Sciences; a Contribution to a New Scientific Ideal.* Trans. from the Dutch by Henry J. Koren. (Duquesne Studies, Psychological Series, 1) Pittsburgh, Duquesne University Press, 1963, pp. 3-9.

2. In this country, the technical term "behavior" applies to human and animal behavior; in the European literature, the term "behavior" and its equivalents in other languages, e.g., *comportement* in French, *Verhalten* in German, used to be applied chiefly to the study of animal behavior. This is one reason why, until recently, the term "human sciences" for the study of human behavior was preferred in Europe, and "behavioral sciences," in this country. These differences appear to be diminishing. Both terms have gained acceptance in the international literature in this field. For a discussion of the varying definitions and the history of these concepts see Ilse Bry and Lois Afflerbach, "In Search of an Organizing Principle for the Behavioral Science Literature," adapted from the authors' editorial in the *Mental Health Book Review Index,* vol. 10, 1965, *Community Mental Health Journal,* February 1968. Cf. Ilse Bry, "Bibliographic Issues in the Behavioral Sciences," in *International Encyclopedia of the Social Sciences.* New York, Macmillan-Free Press, 1968. See also below, note 43.

3. Bernard Berelson and Gary Albert Steiner. *Human Behavior; an Inventory of Scientific Findings.* New York, Harcourt, Brace & World, 1964, p. 11. For other surveys of developments in the behavioral sciences see Rollo Handy and Paul W. Kurtz. *A Current Appraisal of the Behavioral Sciences.* (Behavioral Research Council Bulletin) Great Barrington, Mass., Behavioral Research Council for Scientific Inquiry into the Problems of Men in Society, 1964, and Dan Bergen. "Bibliographic Organization . . . in the Social Sciences." *Wilson Library Bulletin,* vol. 40, April 1966, pp. 751-758.

4. For a comprehensive discussion of the humanities and their contemporary bibliographic resources see Conrad H. Rawski. "Bibliographic Organization . . . in the Humanities." *Wilson Library Bulletin,* vol. 40, April 1966, pp. 738-750. For a discussion of the relations between the behavioral sciences and history, not covered in the present article, see the editorial: "Bibliographic Foundations for an Emergent History of the Behavioral Sciences," *Mental Health Book Review Index,* vol. 12, 1967, pp. i-viii.

5. See, for example, Norman Kiell. *Psychoanalysis, Psychology, and Literature; a Bibliography.* Madison, University of Wisconsin Press, 1963. 4460 references. Norman Kiell. *Psychiatry and Psychology in*

*the Visual Arts and Aesthetics; a Bibliography.* Madison, University of Wisconsin Press, 1965. 7,208 references. See also the journals *American Imago; Journal of Analytical Psychology; Literature and Psychology;* and *Psychoanalytic Review.*

6. This is part of the more general problem discussed in the literature about "science and the humanities." Writings about this topic are relevant as background material to the present article, but cannot be reviewed here. These writings are so scattered and often elusive that no comprehensive bibliography exists. For two succinct presentations of important issues and their history from antiquity to the present, see Max I. Baym. "Science and Poetry," in *Encyclopedia of Poetry and Poetics,* ed. by Alex Preminger. Princeton, Princeton University Press, 1965, pp. 742-753, and *Mental Health Book Review Index,* Editorial Committee. "Changes in the Concept of 'Scientific Literature.' " *Mental Health Book Review Index,* vol. 8, 1963, pp. i-iv; reprinted in *College and Research Libraries,* vol. 25, January 1964, pp. 27-31; expanded with references and notes by Ilse Bry and Lois Afflerbach in *Journal of the History of the Behavioral Sciences,* vol. 1, July 1965, pp. 235-243.

7. *Mental Health Book Review Index; an Annual Bibliography of Books and Book Reviews in the Behavioral Sciences.* Comp. by the Editorial Committee (Ilse Bry, chairman, and Lois Afflerbach, co-chairman) and Contributing Librarians. Flushing, N.Y., Council on Research in Bibliography. Vols. 1-17, 1956-1972.

8. See Ruth Nanda Anshen, below, note 73. p. 7.

9. Sigmund Freud, *Delusions and Dreams in Jensen's* Gradiva, in *The Standard Edition of the Complete Psychological Works of Sigmund Freud.* Trans. and ed. by James Strachey. Vol. 9. New York, Macmillan, 1959, pp. 1-95; espec. p. 8.

10. Arthur Koestler. *The Act of Creation.* Foreword by Sir Cyril Burt. New York, Macmillan, 1964, p. 18.

11. Warren G. Bennis *et al. Interpersonal Dynamics; Essays and Readings on Human Interaction.* Foreword by Douglas McGregor. (The Dorsey Series in Psychology) Homewood, Ill., Dorsey Press, 1964. Foreword, p. vi; Preface, p. x; p. 2, p. 220.

12. Sylvia Brody. *Passivity, a Study of Its Development and Expression in Boys.* New York, International Universities Press, 1964. Appendix: "Footnotes from Literature," pp. 156-172.

13. Jan Hendrick van den Berg. *The Changing Nature of Man; Introduction to a Historical Psychology (Metabletica).* Trans. from the Dutch by H. F. Croes. New York, Norton, 1961, pp. 26, 71-72. Paperback edition: New York, Delta, Dell, 1964. (A Delta Book, 1162)

14. Child Study Association of America. *A Reader for Parents; a Selection of Creative Literature about Childhood,* ed. by Anna W. M. Wolf. New York, Norton, 1963. Introduction, p. 12.

15. Erving Goffman. *Stigma; Notes on the Management of Spoiled Identity.* Englewood Cliffs, N.J., Prentice-Hall, 1963, p. 112. Also published as paperback: (A Spectrum Book, S-73)

16. Margaret Phillips. *Small Social Groups in England.* London, Methuen, 1965, p. 4. "A Sociologist's Footnote," by Bryan Wilson, p. 303.

17. Norman Kiell, ed. *The Universal Experience of Adolescence.* New York, International Universities Press, 1964, p. 9. Bibliography, pp. 884-942.

18. Carney Landis. *Varieties of Psychopathological Experience,* ed. by Fred A. Mettler. New York, Holt, Rinehart and Winston, 1964.

19. Bert Kaplan, ed. *The Inner World of Mental Illness: A Series of First-Person Accounts of What It Was Like.* New York, Harper and Row, 1964.

20. See Child Study Association of America, above, note 14; Norman Kiell, above, note 17; I. D. Harris, below, note 29.

21. Clifford Whittingham Beers. *A Mind That Found Itself; an Autobiography.* New York, Longmans, Green, 1908. 5th ed. rev., Garden City, N.Y. Doubleday, 1956.

22. William Ellery Leonard. *The Locomotive-God.* New York, Century, 1927.

23. Morag Coate, *pseud. Beyond All Reason.* With an Introduction by R. D. Laing. Philadelphia, Lippincott, 1965, pp. vii-viii. See also Laing and Esterson, below, note 59.

24. Sarah E. Lorenz, *pseud. And Always Tomorrow.* New York, Holt, Rinehart and Winston, 1963.

25. Christoph Haizmann, died 1700. *Schizophrenia 1677; a Psychiatric Study of an Illustrated Autobiographical Record of Demoniacal Possession,* by Ida Macalpine and Richard A. Hunter. (Psychiatric Monograph Series, no. 2) London, Dawson, 1956. With a translation (pp. 57-85) and reproduction (pp. 167-191) of Manuscript 14.084, National-Bibliothek, Vienna.

26. Kurt Robert Eissler. *Goethe: A Psychoanalytic Study, 1775-1786.* 2 vols. Detroit, Wayne State University Press, 1963.

27. Phyllis Greenacre. *The Quest for the Father; a Study of the Darwin-Butler Controversy, as a Contribution to the Understanding of the Creative Individual.* (The Freud Anniversary Lecture Series of the New York Psychoanalytic Institute, 1962) New York, International Universities Press, 1963.

28. Ian Macfarlane Smith. *Spatial Ability: Its Educational and Social Significance.* San Diego, Calif., Knapp, 1964. Appendixes, pp. 302-351, espec. p. 315.

29. Irving David Harris. *The Promised Seed; a Comparative Study of Eminent First and Later Sons.* New York, Free Press of Glencoe, 1964.

30. Victor Goertzel and Mildred George Goertzel. *Cradles of Eminence.* Boston, Little, Brown, 1962, p. 272.

31. Julius Ernst Heuscher. *A Psychiatric Study of Fairy Tales: Their Origin, Meaning, and Usefulness.* Springfield, Ill., Thomas, 1963, pp. 6, 189-198. Bibliography, pp. 213-215. List of Fairy Tales and Myths Mentioned in the Text, pp. 217-218.

32. Evelyn Goodenough Pitcher and Ernst Prelinger. *Children Tell Stories; an Analysis of Fantasy.* Foreword by Margaret Lowenfeld. New York, International Universities Press, 1963, pp. 8, 240.

33. Arthur Koestler, above, note 10.

34. See Norman Kiell, above, note 5.

35. Frank Xavier Barron. *Creativity and Psychological Health; Origins of Personal Vitality and Creative Freedom.* Princeton, Van Nostrand, 1963, pp. 242-243.

36. Ellis Paul Torrance. *Guiding Creative Talent.* Englewood Cliffs, N.J., Prentice-Hall, 1962, p. 116.

37. Dale Benner Harris. *Children's Drawings as Measures of Intellectual Maturity; a Revision and Extension of the Goodenough Draw-a-Man Test.* New York, Harcourt, Brace & World, 1963. Chapter 2: "Historical Survey of the Study of Children's Drawings," pp. 10-36, espec. pp. 12-13.

38. See Norman Kiell, above, note 5.

39. Joseph Szigeti. "Composer, Performer, and Audience," in Seymour Morgan Farber and Roger H. L. Wilson, eds. *Man and Civilization: Conflict and Creativity; a Symposium.* New York, McGraw-Hill, 1963, pp. 303-314, espec. p. 313. Also published as paperback.

40. Christoph Haizmann, above, note 25, p. 6.

41. Margaret Mead and Martha Wolfenstein, eds. *Childhood in Contemporary Cultures.* Chicago, University of Chicago Press, 1955, pp. 229-293, espec. p. 235. Also published as paperback, 1963. (Phoenix Books, P124)

42. See also the *Journal of Creative Behavior* and the bibliographical and indexing journal *Perceptual-Cognitive Development.*

43. From the definition of the behavioral sciences suggested in 1960 in an editorial of the *Mental Health Book Review Index* (vol. 5, no. 1), "The Behavioral Sciences and Mental Health in Relation to the Organization of Knowledge, the Organization of Science, and Bibliography":

"A composite of those interpretations of the term which agree on the scientific goal, man's understanding of himself, suggests a tentative definition of the *behavioral sciences* as a multidisciplinary pursuit of knowledge about behavior in its roots and manifestations, in man and animals, in individuals, groups, and cultures, and in all conditions, normal, exceptional, and pathological." Reprinted as editorial in *A.M.A. Archives of General Psychiatry*, vol. 2, June 1960, pp. 701-706, espec. p. 701.

44. Joseph Church. *Language and the Discovery of Reality; a Developmental Psychology of Cognition.* New York. Random House, 1961. Paperback edition: New York, Vintage Books, 1966. (A Vintage Book V338). Heinz Werner and Bernard Kaplan. *Symbol Formation; an Organismic-Developmental Approach to Language and the Expression of Thought.* New York, Wiley, 1963.

45. Aleen Agranowitz and Milfred Riddle McKeown. *Aphasia Handbook for Adults and Children.* Rev. and enl. ed. Springfield, Ill., Thomas, 1964. Hildred Schuell, James J. Jenkins, and Edward Jiménez-Pabón. *Aphasia in Adults: Diagnosis, Prognosis, and Treatment.* New York. Hoeber Medical Division, Harper and Row, 1964.

46. Symposium on Disorders of Language, London, 1963. *Ciba Foundation Symposium: Disorders of Language,* ed. by A. V. S. de Reuck and Maeve O'Connor. Boston, Little, Brown, 1964.

47. Macdonald Critchley. *Developmental Dyslexia.* Springfield, Ill., Thomas, 1964, p. 72.

48. Florence G. Roswell and Gladys Natchez. *Reading Disability: Diagnosis and Treatment.* New York, Basic Books, 1964. pp. 71-72.

49. William F. Fry, Jr. *Sweet Madness: a Study of Humor.* Palo Alto, Calif., Pacific Books, 1963.

50. Jerome Lewis Schulman, Joseph C. Kaspar, and Patricia M. Barger. *The Therapeutic Dialogue: a Method for the Analysis of Verbal Interaction.* Springfield, Ill., Thomas, 1964.

51. Wilbur Lang Schramm, Jack Lyle, and Ithiel de Sola Pool. *The People Look at Educational Television; a Report of Nine Representative ETV Stations.* Stanford, Calif., Stanford University Press, 1963.

52. Charles Aubrey Thomas *et al. Programmed Learning in Perspective; a Guide to Program Writing.* Chicago, Educational Methods, 1965.

53. See also *British Journal of Disorders of Communication* (incorporating *Speech Pathology and Therapy*); *Journal of Reading; Journal of Speech and Hearing Disorders; Journal of Speech and Hearing Research; Language and Speech; Programmed Learning; Reading Improvement; Reading Teacher;* and the now discontinued journal *Logos.*

54. Henri Baruk, *Hebraic Civilization and the Science of Man.* Trans. from the French by Philip Polack. (Mary Hemingway Rees Memorial Lecture. 2d. 1960. A World Mental Health Year Publication) London, World Federation for Mental Health, 1961.

55. Hans Jacobs. *Western Psychotherapy and Hindu-Ŝâdhanâ: a Contribution to Comparative Studies in Psychology and Metaphysics.* New York. International Universities Press, 1961.

56. Joseph Lyons. *Psychology and the Measure of Man: a Phenomenological Approach.* New York. Free Press of Glencoe, 1963. Preface, pp. ix-x; pp. 5-29.

57. Igor Alexander Caruso. *Existential Psychology: from Analysis to Synthesis.* Trans. from the German by Eva Krapf. New York. Herder and Herder, 1964.

58. Stephen Strasser, above, note 1.

59. Ronald David Laing and A. Esterson. *Sanity, Madness, and the Family. Vol. 1: Families of Schizophrenics.* (Studies in Existential Analysis and Phenomenology) London, Tavistock, 1964; New York, Basic Books, 1965. See also Morag Coate, *pseud.*, above, note 23.

60. Trenton William Wann, ed. *Behaviorism and Phenomenology; Contrasting Bases for Modern Psychology.* (Rice University Semicentennial Publications) Chicago, Published for William Marsh Rice University by the University of Chicago Press, 1964. Introduction, p. viii. Also published as paperback, 1965. (Phoenix Books, P. 192).

61. According to James E. Dittes, perhaps 1,000 papers are written annually in the general field of the scientific study of religion. Cf. "Editorial Foreword," *Journal for the Scientific Study of Religion,* vol. 6, April 1967, p. 2.

62. See William Douglas, below, note 64.

63. Margaretta K. Bowers. *Conflicts of the Clergy; a Psychodynamic Study with Case Histories.* New York, Nelson, 1963. Margaretta K. Bowers *et al. Counseling the Dying.* New York, Nelson, 1964.

64. See Berelson and Steiner, above, note 3.

65. William Douglas. "Religion." in Norman Louis Farberow, ed. *Taboo Topics.* (The Atherton Press Behavioral Science Series) New York, Atherton Press, 1963, pp. 80-95, espec. pp. 82-84. Selected Bibliography, pp. 93-95. Also published as paperback, 1966. (An Atheling Book, SP-506).

66. Michael Argyle. *Religious Behavior.* Glencoe, Ill., Free Press, 1959. Preface, p. xi.

67. Samuel Zundel Klausner. *Psychiatry and Religion.* New York, Free Press of Glencoe, 1964, espec. pp. 5, 8, 20. Bibliography, pp. 281-299.

68. Mircea Eliade. *Shamanism: Archaic Techniques of Ecstasy.* Trans. from the French by Willard R. Trask. Rev. and enl. ed. (Bollingen Series, 76) New York, Bollingen Foundation; Pantheon Books, 1964. Foreword, pp. xi, xx.

69. Ari Kiev, ed. *Magic, Faith, and Healing; Studies in Primitive Psychiatry Today.* New York, Free Press of Glencoe, 1964.

70. Abraham Harold Maslow. *Religions, Values, and Peak Experiences.* (The Kappa Delta Pi Lecture Series, vol. 35) Columbus, Ohio State University Press, 1964. Preface, pp. xii, xv; pp. 19-20, 57.

71. Milton Rokeach. *The Three Christs of Ypsilanti: a Psychological Study.* New York, Knopf, 1964. Paperback edition: New York, Vintage Books, 1967. (A Vintage Book, V395)

72. See also the journals *Insight: Quarterly Review of Religion and Mental Health; Journal of Pastoral Care; Journal of Religion and Health; Journal for the Scientific Study of Religion; Pastoral Counselor; Pastoral Psychology; Review of Religious Research;* and the series, "The Dwight Harrington Terry Foundation Lectures on Religion in the Light of Science and Philosophy," e.g., vol. 34: Margaret Mead, *Continuities in Cultural Evolution.* New Haven, Yale University Press, 1964.

73. Ruth Nanda Anshen. "Religious Perspectives: Its Meaning and Purpose," in Erich Fromm. *The Heart of Man, Its Genius for Good and Evil.* (Religious Perspectives, vol. 12) New York, Harper and Row, 1964, pp. 7-11. The series editor also expresses the hope "that the rediscovery of man will point the way to the rediscovery of God." p. 7.

74. See Mircea Eliade, above, note 68. Foreword, p. xv.

75. Richard Hosmer Blum and Associates. *Utopiates; the Use and Users of LSD 25.* (The Atherton Press Behavioral Science Series) New York, Atherton Press, 1964. Sidney Cohen. *The Beyond Within; the LSD Story.* New York, Atheneum, 1964. Timothy Francis Leary, Ralph Metzner, and Richard Alpert. *The Psychedelic Experience; a Manual Based on the Tibetan Book of the Dead.* (Psychedelic Monograph 1) New Hyde Park, N.Y., University Books, 1964. David Solomon, ed. *LSD: the Consciousness-Expanding Drug.* New York, Putnam, 1964. Also issued as paperback, 1966. (A Berkeley Medallion Book, N1277) See also the journal *Psychedelic Review.*

76. In addition to the journals already mentioned, see also *Educational Theory; Etc.: a Review of General Semantics; Inquiry; Journal of Humanistic Psychology; Studies in Philosophy and Education;* and *Systematics.*

77. Daniel Casriel. *So Fair a House; the Story of Synanon.* (Human and Social Behavior) Englewood Cliffs, N.J., Prentice-Hall, 1963.

78. Jack Harold Kahn and Jean P. Nursten. *Unwillingly to School;*

*the Place of the Child Guidance Clinic in the Treatment of School Phobia.* (The Commonwealth and International Library. Mental Health and Social Medicine Division, vol. 1) New York, Macmillan, 1964.

79. William F. Fry, Jr., above, note 49.

80. I. D. Harris, above, note 29.

81. George Morris Carstairs. *This Island Now; the Surge of Social Change in the Twentieth Century.* (The B. B. C. Reith Lectures, 1962) New York, Basic Books. 1962. Introduction, p. 10.

82. W. H. Auden. *Look Stranger!* London, Faber and Faber, 1936. p. 19. American edition with title: *On This Island.* New York, Random House, 1937, p. 19.

# ESSAY 10

## *Bibliographic Foundations for an Emergent History of the Behavioral Sciences*

Originally published as Editorial in *Mental Health Book Review Index,* vol. 12 (whole no. 17), 1967.

There are few basic concepts in the history of ideas that have changed their meaning as radically as has the concept of history itself. Traditionally, historical studies were limited to political and military events and involved a probing into a past not witnessed by the generation alive at the time of its writing. Beginning in the 19th century, the history of culture, of ideas, and of science became new fields of specialization. The historian's insistence on a long perspective began to yield in the first half of the 20th century, when continual crises called for immediate analysis through work in contemporary history. The period during which the field of history was modified in these two ways is the same that saw the advent of the behavioral sciences. New perspectives then opened with the rise of social history and a merging of historical and psychological concerns. Arthur O. Lovejoy, one of the founders of intellectual history as a discipline, closed his essay on "The Historiography of Ideas" (1938) by referring to this field as "the endeavor to investigate the history, and thereby, it may be hoped, to understand better the nature, of the workings of the human mind."

### A NEW PHASE IN THE HISTORY OF HISTORY

It has been left to the second half of the 20th century to investigate the history of the endeavor directly concerned with studying the human mind and the whole range of human nature, relations, and affairs. To help envision this new phase, this essay will attempt to point out the variety of contributions that are being made toward a history of the behavioral sciences. In the light of research in bibliography, it will also touch on other developments in this area that have historical implications. Although the concept "behavioral science" was introduced only about 1950,[1] the various approaches to the scientific study of man made since the mid-19th century can now be seen as the emergent behavioral sciences, unified in retrospect. The *Journal of the History of the Behavioral Sciences,* launched in 1963, reflects and reinforces this trend. Among the obstacles to writing the history of the behavioral sciences as a broad intellectual movement have been specialization within separate disciplines, emphasis on recent advances at the expense of background knowledge, and neglect of primary sources. Interest in work of a historical nature, even if limited in scope, has, however, grown in this whole area during the past ten years.

## HISTORY OF DISCIPLINES—RISE AND TRANSITION

A concern of behavioral scientists with the history of their own disciplines is the most tangible of the new trends. For example, Paul Bohannan notes "an absolute rash of anthropological history-mongering in the last few years" in his review of three anthropological books that trace "The Making of a Social Science" (*Science,* 26 May 1967, pp. 1076-1077). Also in the 1960s, a Division for the History of Psychology was formed in the American Psychological Association, and the Archives of the History of American Psychology were founded at the University of Akron.

In the psychological sciences, changing attitudes are markedly involved in this quest for background orientation. In the early 1950s, the psychiatrist Leo Kanner raised the question of whether a competent specialist needed to know the antecedents in his profession.[2] He then tried to test how well his colleagues in the younger generation were informed about the contributions to their field made by fifteen men in the late 19th and early 20th centuries. The nearly 300 respondents to his questionnaire showed little pertinent knowledge or even interest. For example, in one hundred of their answers they identified such a notable contributor to psychiatry not in terms of his own work, but merely—and even this often wrongly—as a forerunner, teacher, contemporary, co-worker, supporter, or opponent of Freud, or simply by "the all-important word 'pre-Freud.' " At that time, Kanner found the *History of Medical Psychology* by Zilboorg and Henry, published in 1941, to be virtually the only major source for background information. Since the mid-1950s, however, a dozen more or less extensive histories of psychiatry and psychotherapy have been published and discussed in the review literature.

For the history of psychoanalysis, the Freud centenary year, 1956, seems to have been a turning point. A tendency to reiterate legends and controversies that had surrounded Freud's life and work for half a century has since given way to concern with a broader and more objective record.[3] Three volumes of Freud's previously unpublished correspondence[4] and the *Minutes of the Vienna Psychoanalytic Society*[5] provide new source material. Selected papers of many authors who have further contributed to psychoanalysis are now available in book form. Collected papers, letters, and posthumous works of those who, like Adler, Burrow, Sullivan, Clara Thompson, and others, represent different schools of thought, also appeared during this time. Biographies combined with evaluation have lately tried to do justice to less known figures such as Groddeck[6] and forty other "psychoanalytic pioneers." A recent book with this title[7] extends the concept of pioneer from the early days of psychoanalysis to the present, suggesting the emergence of a contemporary history of science.

Studies and textbooks in the history of psychology have also increased in number. They remain separate from those in psychiatry and psychoanalysis, although sometimes there is more overlapping in the content of all these books than is apparent from their auspices, titles, and use. Freud is claimed for the history of each of the three disciplines. Another common tendency is to push the background beyond the limits of a 19th-century discipline and even of modern science to the origin of Western civilization and still farther back to prehistoric times.[8] The next step, and one that is crucial for a true perspective on the sciences of man, would be a unified history of the psychological sciences.

## CONTRIBUTIONS TO CULTURAL, SOCIAL, AND INTELLECTUAL HISTORY

Historical work in several branches of the behavioral sciences has blended with the history of culture, as suggested in the title of one book, "Greek Culture and the Ego,"[9] the subtitle of another, "a psycho-historical theory of culture based on relations between the arts, psychology, and the social sciences,"[10] and the works on the history of insanity by Foucault[11] and Leibbrand and Wettley.[12] Certain movements which form part of social and cultural history also fall within the area of the behavioral sciences, for example, those relating to capital punishment and penal reform, abortion and contraception, addiction and homosexuality. The relevance of socio-historical contributions to current writings and concerns is suggested in a study of America's awakening to poverty as a social problem, c. 1830-1925, published in 1956.[13] The author notes that "in every generation [earnest critics] have reminded us that poverty is shameful . . . to the society that allows it to exist." Topics chosen to trace the evolution of thought range from specific concepts like the unconscious and instinctive behavior to major theories like ego psychology. Some ideas now important for the intellectual history of the behavioral sciences have had their origin in other fields. For example, it is possible to trace through this literature the absorption of existentialism, at first only a philosophical movement, by psychology, psychiatry, and psychoanalysis.

The review literature, which brings into focus work of special interest to the scientific community, reveals also the rise of ideas not yet studied in historical perspective. One of them is the concept of change. Changing attitudes of individuals and groups, change of behavior as a therapeutic goal, the facts and impact of social and technological change, measurement and strategies of change, change observed, planned, or manipulated, the changing outlook in professional work and subject fields, biological change and change in Western civilization and the nature of man—all of these seemingly diverse approaches might be considered together in a historical study of "change" as a basic conceptual orientation for behavioral scientists.

## PRIMARY SOURCES, PERIODS OF TIME, AND THE HISTORICAL THRESHOLD

The adoption of historical methods in the behavioral sciences has encouraged an approach through original sources, which was previously seldom used. Many virtually inaccessible documents have been made available for wider study. Some of these illustrate the evolution of thought. Examples are a history of psychiatry presented in selected English texts, 1535-1860, and some early contributions to psychosomatic medicine and forensic psychiatry which have recently been republished.[14] Several source books in the history of psychology serve the same purpose.[15] In other instances, new knowledge has been sought in previously unpublished documents. Chenevix-Trench consulted the private diaries of two of King George III's physicians for an account of his insanity in 1788-1789.[16] Josef and Renée Gicklhorn studied 5,000 pieces of archival material at the University of Vienna, forty of which they published in their book on Sigmund Freud's academic career in light of the documents.[17] An exhaustive use of primary sources forms the basis for a social and psychological history of a German prison camp, Ruhleben, where John Davidson Ketchum had himself been interned during the First World War.[18] He continued almost to the end of his life in 1962 to obtain additional source material from other ex-prisoners so that his book suggests a transition from the study of existing to the creation of new historical sources through questionnaires, interviews, and other instruments of social science research. Interviews held with Jung in 1957, filmed and later published by Richard I. Evans,[19] are an early example of the production of source material now widely practiced as "oral history."

For the historical periods studied, "anniversary" years from 25 to 200 tend to be favored. In the late 1950s, the past fifty years became significant for the behavioral sciences. Important pioneer work done prior to World War I, and then dormant for varying intervals, aroused new interest in a new context after World War II. Examples are the revival of the mental hygiene movement in the form of the contemporary, worldwide movement for mental health, the renewed application of the pedagogic methods of Maria Montessori, and the recent concern with the child-rearing practices of the kibbutz in Israel.[20] A number of studies in social history cover time spans from the middle of one to the middle of the next or second next century, suggesting that socially significant periods cut across rather than stay within the centuries that govern the customary chronological breakdown in the humanities.[21] Variations in the length of time covered and in its distance from the present reflect the changing pace of developments seen in historical perspective.[22] If it could be ascertained how fast a given field moves toward its historical threshold, it might be possible to predict when pioneer work is apt to be retrieved from temporary oblivion and restored to the historical record, perhaps even rediscovered as a stimulus to current research.

## INDIRECT HISTORICAL CONTRIBUTIONS

Observance of actual anniversaries, especially centennials of institutions and of men like Darwin and Freud, and birthdays of the older behavioral scientists, has led to a growing literature of Festschriften. A now popular variant type of "Festschrift" first takes the form of a conference, and this return to the spoken symposium applies also to memorial observances and centennial celebrations. The need to evaluate the resulting publications is today more recognized than before. At its best, this form of scientific literature recaptures through creative editorship a life-long process of intellectual integration. Its study may, therefore, lead to a better understanding of the forces that help shape the history of ideas. In various other fields, Festschriften, which have a history of a hundred years, gained in the mid-20th century the recognition of bibliographers, whose primary intent then was to index the individual articles that had previously been lost to the record of a discipline or subject field. A future bibliography of Festschriften in the behavioral sciences should also try to bring out the dynamic interrelationships that make a Festschrift distinctive and unique.

In 1924, the then retired Director-General of the Prussian State Library, better known as the theologian Adolf von Harnack, published "a bibliographic suggestion" concerning book dedications.[23] He proposed that dedications, other than those to the author's family, be added to the cataloging of current and older books. Von Harnack used illustrations from the oldest Christian literature to show that the extant dedications, even of works that are themselves lost, throw new light on the relationships between pagan and Christian authors or between representatives of Christian faith and secular power. From these studies he concluded that the historical value of dedications may outlast that of the books.

Dedications found in the literature of the behavioral sciences now seem to be taking on historical significance. In the absence of bibliographic data for the past, it is hard to tell whether it was then an exception that Edwin G. Boring, one of the most history-minded American psychologists, dedicated two of his works in the history of psychology to Titchener (1929) and Helmholtz (1942). The *Mental Health Book Review Index* began in 1965 to record professionally meaningful dedications, and with the present Volume 12, 1967, this policy has been fully adopted. Fifty-five dedications, two-thirds of which appear in the present volume of the *Index*, have been noted so far. For a transdisciplinary history of the behavioral sciences, it may be of interest that the names include the anthropologist Bronislaw Malinowski, the criminologist Hermann Mannheim, the sociologist Ernest Watson Burgess, the educator James B. Conant, the neuroscientists W. Horsley Gantt and H. W. Magoun, the psychologists Carl I. Hovland, David Rapaport, and L. L. Thurstone, the psychiatrists Gerald Caplan, Roy R. Grinker, Sr., and J. Wolpe, the psychoanalysts Frieda Fromm-Reichmann and Heinz Hartmann, the pioneer in animal-behavior and sex research, Robert Mearns Yerkes, the medical historian Henry E. Sigerist, the poet Aldous Huxley, and the philosopher Maurice Merleau-Ponty. As a key to pioneer work, dedications may be even more valuable when the persons are less well known, but their contributions are spelled out in the books. For example, in his preface to *Primate Behavior,*[24] the editor, Irven DeVore, credits Clarence Ray Carpenter, to whom the book is dedicated, with the first field studies of monkeys in 1931, almost twenty-five years before primate research in its current sense became established.

Collections of readings, which have multiplied in recent years, have come under sharp attack, mainly as needless duplication of articles already published in journals. In a letter to the Editor of *Contemporary Psychology* (1967, 12, 286), Leigh Marlowe has gone so far as to suggest to his fellow teachers in psychology that they should never order books of readings for their college library, never use them in courses or reference lists, even write letters to journal editors discouraging their being reviewed. Such a sweeping condemnation, which raises the specter of "bibliocide," misses the point that the best of these "readers" contribute to the history of ideas and draw current attention to writings perhaps at first overlooked. The earliest paper included sometimes antedates by several decades the steady stream of articles that appear when the study of the subject has become popular. An example of collected readings that amount to a topical history is *The Nature of Hypnosis* by Shor and Orne.[25] The articles and excerpts from books published from 1784 to 1963 are supplemented by a selected bibliography on the history of hypnotism. Recent volumes of the *Index* try to encourage a careful evaluation of these collections and to suggest the depth of historical approach by giving the inclusive dates of the papers as originally published.

Collected papers of individual authors are seldom challenged as a contribution to the history of the behavioral sciences. About fifty of these volumes have been listed in the *Index*. The authors include, besides the psychoanalysts already mentioned, Boring,[26] Lashley,[27] Whorf,[28] and others in a variety of fields. More complete, but also more elusive, than these selections are the bibliographies of the authors' writings. They may be appended to the selected papers, to Festschriften, to the monographs in a lecture series, to critical essays, or simply to a book whose author wants to put his complete bibliography in print.[29] The inclusive dates tend to span four decades or more, whereas the topical readers, as a rule, cover about twenty years prior to the book's publication.

The author of a scientific book contributes to the continuity of knowledge when he reviews the history of his subject. Freud did so in a masterly fashion in his first major book, *The Interpretation of Dreams* (1900), and was highly praised for it by the contemporary reviewers. German treatises which include a topical history may still mention the word *Geschichte* in the title, but the titles of current American and British books are not so explicit. The *Index* now indicates whether books contain reviews of the literature and also points out material of historical interest that may be a feature of the book, often in the form of appendixes. Examples are the history of nudity and nudism in Western civilization with which Fred Ilfeld, Jr. and Roger Lauer introduce their social-psychological study of present-day *Social Nudism in America*,[30] a review of the psychiatric nosologies of all times, appended to Karl Menninger's *The Vital Balance*,[31] and Kurt Eissler's rebuttal[32] of the book by the Gicklhorns on Freud mentioned earlier.

## HISTORIOGRAPHY AND BIBLIOGRAPHY

Entirely different approaches are involved in tracing the evolution of theories and concepts or the history of organizations and of institutions such as prisons and psychiatric hospitals, in editing personal documents such as letters or conducting initial archival research. The *Index,* as a continuous bibliography that contains examples of virtually all kinds of historical studies pertinent to the behavioral sciences, may help to develop a historiography of the field. The attitude toward keeping records for the historian of the future has also varied greatly in different periods and places. In recent years the preserving of original records has become a preoccupation of a growing number of behavioral scientists.

History rests, however, not only on documents as such, but on the historian's ability to recognize and interpret what is significant. Moreover, basic records can be lost without being physically destroyed. For a history of the emergent behavioral sciences in the late 19th and early 20th centuries, the decisive loss was the break in intellectual continuity caused by the First World War. The vast periodical and bibliographic literature which, until then, had served the scientists and scholars in this area in their international and interdisciplinary relationships suffered a severe setback, and much of it was later neither revived nor remembered.[33] A fruitful contribution to a comprehensive history of the behavioral sciences might be made in the form of bibliographic guides to this buried European and American literature, and through developing competence and interest in library research with now unknown and unsuspected printed sources.

## ISSUES AND OUTLOOK

Can there be a history of the behavioral sciences while they continue to lack a tangible identity? The behavioral sciences have neither achieved nor sought unity in terms of scientific organization. Scientists identified with this area function under the auspices available to them which, whether disciplinary or interdisciplinary, old or new, are necessarily specialized. The contrast to medicine is noteworthy. The history of medicine was favored at an early date by the initial unity of the field and, as Kanner suggested, the history of the specialties into which medicine was gradually subdivided has been lagging behind. In the behavioral sciences, the lack of organizational unity and the continuing emphasis on the history of each specialty has retarded the inception, even the conception, of a unified history.

It cannot be denied, however, that the behavioral sciences have been organizing themselves in their own way. Their form of organization is functional rather than structural, invisible rather than conspicuous, mobile rather than static, in other words, adapted to the 20th century to which they belong. This development is of historical interest. As far as possible, the *Index* has, therefore, noted the auspices under which work was done, furthered, or published. This includes matters pertaining to scientific organization within the literature such as monographic series, lectureships, patterns of publishing and distribution in more than one country, and the thesis on which some of these books are based. For example, Amacher's study of the neurological views of Freud's teachers and their influence on his early psychoanalytic writings[34] began as a doctoral dissertation in history, a bibliographic detail that suggests that the rapprochement between the behavioral sciences and history may be or become mutual. The review literature may also help those who try to see the interdisciplinary composition of the behavioral sciences not as being settled by one or the other definition, but rather as an ongoing historical process. Schaller's book, *The Mountain Gorilla; Ecology and Behavior,*[35] for example, was reviewed in *Animal Behaviour* in 1963, in *Human Biology* in 1964, in *Contemporary Psychology* in 1965, and in the *American Journal of Sociology* in 1966.

Finally, has there been a new, direct confrontation between the behavioral sciences and history in the general sense and, if so, can this be traced through bibliographic data? Although history as a discipline has moved from the humanities to the social sciences, there are inherent conflicts, especially with the psychological sciences. Attempts to offer psychological, in particular psychoanalytic, interpretations of historical figures have often been severely criticized. Moreover, to be historic in the traditional sense, an event must be significant for society as a whole. The concept of "history" intrinsic to psychology applies, however, to personal, especially clinical data about individuals and groups, and a whole book may be devoted to the case history of one child. Certain topics of special concern to one discipline appear to have met with rejection by the other. For example, in *The History of Prostitution,*

Bullough[36] points out that prostitution has been "almost a taboo topic for the professional historian," and the book *Taboo Topics,* edited by Farberow,[37] contains a chapter on the psychologist in international affairs.

Nevertheless, the outlook has been changing. In 1932, it was Einstein who posed the question, "Is there any way of delivering mankind from the menace of war?", to Freud, who was taken by surprise and "dumbfounded by the thought of [his own] incompetence," this being "the statesman's proper study."[38] Now many behavioral scientists are raising the same question, and even though the answer seems as remote as it is urgent, the specialists concerned have taken up various other psychological, social, psychiatric, and global issues relating to war, from concentration camps and "brainwashing" to radiation and world politics. A collection of classical and contemporary writings by psychologists, sociologists, and anthropologists on the causes of war, which inincludes the famous essay by William James written before World War I as well as Freud's answer to Einstein. "Why War?", written before World War II, covers almost a hundred years.[39] While history as a field has been refined by moving from a preoccupation with military affairs to the study of ideas, similar progress in the behavioral sciences has led to an increasing concern with the problems and the prevention of war.

A broadening of the common ground between historians and behavioral scientists is further illustrated by the response of psychologists and psychiatrists to the Kennedy administration and to the assassination. Four books, two on mental retardation, one on physical fitness, and one on *Acting Out,* are dedicated to John Fitzgerald Kennedy, the last citing him as the "35th President of the United States who stood for reason and intelligence in human affairs and became the victim of acting out destructiveness."[40] A revised edition of Walter Bromberg's *Crime and the Mind,* published in 1965, includes a case history of Jack Ruby, who was then still living.[41] *Children and the Death of a President,* a collection of studies edited by Martha Wolfenstein and Gilbert Kliman,[42] makes some of the saliènt points explicit. The editors stress that they speak as social scientists rather than as historians, yet they regard these studies in part as "historical documents of the immediate meaning of a major national event to those who experienced it" and point out that child experts "have here widened their scope to see their subjects in a national context." Furthermore, they report that thirty-nine studies of reactions to the assassination of President Kennedy had been listed by April 1964, and link the practical urgency of such disaster research with the possibility of a future nuclear war.

It is still a long way from an awakening sense of historical perspectives to a plan for an integrated history of the behavioral sciences. The efforts here surveyed, from disciplinary and topical historical studies to an active participation in historical processes, are diverse, diffuse, and as yet undirected. What matters most, however, is the growing readiness among behavioral scientists to transcend limits too narrowly drawn and to relate a fair share of specialized work about human behavior to the ultimate issues of man's continued existence. It is this transcending commitment that may draw historians and behavioral scientists together in a common task. History has lent its method to give the behavioral sciences a past. The behavioral sciences, in their concern with planning for what is desired, preventing what is feared, may help history to extend its horizon, even beyond the present, to mankind's ever more foreseeable future.

## REFERENCES AND NOTES

1. For a discussion of different definitions of the term "behavioral sciences" and further references *see* the editorial "In Search of an Organizing Principle for the Behavioral Science Literature," p. 69. *See also* Senn, Peter R. "What Is 'Behavioral Science?'–Notes Toward a History." *Journal of the History of the Behavioral Sciences,* 1966, 2, 107-122.

2. Kanner, Leo. "The Status of Historical Perspective in Psychiatric Instruction." *Bulletin of the History of Medicine,* 1955, 29, 329-336.

3. Observations and examples used are largely based on the book literature, roughly for the period from 1955 to 1965, which has been covered in the twelve volumes of the *Mental Health Book Review Index.*

4a. Freud, Sigmund. *Letters of Sigmund Freud.* Selected and ed. by Ernst L. Freud. N.Y., Basic Books, 1960. 470 pp. British ed. with title: *Letters of Sigmund Freud, 1873-1939.* London, Hogarth Press, 1961. 470 pp. Paperback ed.: N.Y., McGraw-Hill, 1964. 470 pp.

4b. Freud, Sigmund, and Pfister, Oskar. *Psycho-analysis and faith; the letters of Sigmund Freud and Oskar Pfister.* Ed. by Heinrich Meng and Ernst L. Freud. Transl. by Eric Mosbacher. [With prefaces by Ernst L. Freud, Heinrich Meng, and Anna Freud.] London, Hogarth ress, 1963. 152 pp. (The International psycho-analytical library no. 9) N.Y., Basic Books, 1964, © 1963. 152 pp.

4c. Freud, Sigmund, and Abraham, Karl. *A psycho-analytic dia-)gue: the letters of Sigmund Freud and Karl Abraham, 1907-1926.* A selection of 367 from the 492 extant letters.] Ed. by Hilda C. .braham and Ernst L. Freud. Transl. by Bernard Marsh and Hilda C. .braham. [Introd. by Edward Glover.] London, Hogarth Press and ıstitute of Psycho-Analysis, 1965; N.Y., Basic Books, 1966, © 1965. 06 pp. (The International psycho-analytical library, no. 68.)

5. Wiener Psychoanalytische Vereinigung. *Minutes of the Vienna 'sychoanalytic Society.* Vol. 1: 1906-1908. Ed. by Herman Nunberg nd Ernst Federn. Transl. by M. Nunberg. N.Y., International Univer-ities Press, 1962. 410 pp.

6. Grossman, Carl Michael, and Grossman, Sylva. *The wild analyst; he life and work of Georg Groddeck.* [Dedicated to the memory of rieda Fromm-Reichmann. With excerpts from the correspondence etween Groddeck and Freud and with a bibliography.] N.Y., Braziller; ondon, Barrie & Rockliff, 1965. 222 pp. Paperback ed.: N.Y., Delta, ell, 1967. 222 pp. (A Delta book, 9542.)

7. Alexander, Franz, Eisenstein, Samuel, and Grotjahn, Martin, ds. *Psychoanalytic pioneers.* [Biographical essays of followers of reud from Karl Abraham to Erik H. Erikson, with evaluations of their ontributions to the evolution of psychoanalytic thought. With chap-ers on psychoanalysis in England and in the United States to the early 960s. With bibliographies.] N.Y., London, Basic Books, 1966. 616 pp.

8a. Alexander, Franz, and Selesnick, Shelton T. *The history of sychiatry; an evaluation of psychiatric thought and practice from pre-istoric times to the present.* [Completed by Sheldon T. Selesnick after ne death of Franz Alexander in March 1964. Dedicated to the mem-ry of Franz Alexander. Introd. by Jules Masserman. With bibliog-aphies.] N.Y., Harper & Row, 1966. 471 pp.

8b. Herrnstein, Richard Julius, and Boring, Edwin Garrigues, eds. *source book in the history of psychology.* [Excerpts from sources, a. 350 B.C. to 1929, partly translated for this book by various trans-ators. Series editor's pref. by Edward H. Madden. With a list of ex-erpted works.] Cambridge, Harvard Univ. Pr.; London, Oxford Univ. r. [distributor], 1965. 636 pp. (Source books in the history of the ciences.)

8c. Watson, Robert Irving. *The great psychologists: from Aristotle ) Freud.* Philadelphia, Lippincott, 1963. 572 pp. Text ed.: Philadel-hia, Lippincott, 1963. 572 pp. (The Lippincott college psychology series.)

9. Stokes, Adrian Durham. *Greek culture and the ego; a psychoanalytic survey of an aspect of Greek civilization and of art.* London, Tavistock, 1958. 101 pp.

10. Abell, Walter. *The collective dream in art; a psycho-historical theory of culture based on relations between the arts, psychology, and the social sciences.* Cambridge, Harvard Univ. Pr.; London, Oxford Univ. Pr., 1957. 378 pp.

11. Foucault, Michel. *Madness and civilization; a history of insanity in the age of reason.* Transl. from the French [Histoire de la folie à l'âge classique; folie et déraison, abridged by the author, Paris, 1964, ©1961] by Richard Howard. [With the author's addition of material from the original edition, Paris, 1961, including the chapter "Passion and Delirium.' Introd. by José Barchilon. With a bibliography.] N.Y., Pantheon Books, 1965, 299 pp.

12. Leibbrand, Werner, and Wettley, Annemarie. *Der Wahnsinn; Geschichte der abendländischen Psychopathologie.* [Outgrowth of academic work at the Münchener Universitäts-Institut für Geschichte der Medizin.] Freiburg, Alber, 1961. 697 pp. (Orbis academicus; Problemgeschichten der Wissenschaft in Dokumenten und Darstellungen. Bd. 2: [Naturwissenschaftliche Reihe] 12.)

13. Bremner, Robert Hamlett. *From the depths; the discovery of poverty in the United States.* N.Y., New York Univ. Pr., 1956. 364 pp.

14a. Hunter, Richard Alfred, and Macalpine, Ida, eds. *Three hundred years of psychiatry, 1535-1860; a history presented in selected English texts.* [Introduced by explanatory notes] N.Y., London Oxford Univ. Pr., 1963. 1107 pp.

14b. Rather, Lelland Joseph. *Mind and body in eighteenth century medicine; a study based on Jerome Gaub's De regimine mentis,* [first published in Latin, Leiden, 1747 and 1763. A new English translation, with an introd., commentaries and notes. With a bibliography.] Berkeley, Univ. of California Pr., 1965. 274 pp. London, Wellcome Historical Medical Library, 1965. 275 pp. (Publications of the Wellcome Historical Medical Library, new ser., vol. 7.)

14c. Ray, Isaac. *A treatise on the medical jurisprudence of insanity.* [The text of the first edition, Boston, 1838. With appendices: Ray's remarks on the McNaughton decision (1843) and the New Hampshire Rule (1869) and "Duties of Medical Witnesses" from the 5th ed., 1871.] Ed. [and with an introd.] by Winfred Overholser. Cambridge, Belknap Press of Harvard Univ. Pr.; London, Oxford Univ. Pr., 1962. 376 pp. (The John Harvard library.)

15a. Herrnstein, Richard Julius, and Boring, Edwin Garrigues, eds. *A source book in the history of psychology.* [Excerpts from sources, ca. 350 B.C. to 1929, partly translated for this book by various translators. Series editor's pref. by Edward H. Madden. With a list of excerpted works.] Cambridge, Harvard Univ. Pr.; London, Oxford Univ. Pr. [distributor], 1965. 636 pp. (Source books in the history of the sciences.)

15b. Shipley, Thorne, ed. *Classics in psychology.* N.Y., Philosophical Library, 1961. 1342 pp.

15c. *Sourcebook in psychology; a course of selected reading by authorities.* Introductory reading guide by James Drever. N.Y., Philosophical Library, 1960. 335 pp.

16. Chenevix-Trench, Charles Pocklington. *The royal malady.* [An account of King George III's attack of insanity in 1788-1789, based on the private, unpublished diaries of two of his physicians, Sir George Baker and Dr. John Willis. With a bibliography.] London, Longmans, 1964; N.Y., Harcourt, Brace & World, 1965, © 1964. 224 pp.

17. Gicklhorn, Josef, and Gicklhorn, Renée. *Sigmund Freuds akademische Laufbahn* [1886-1934] *im Lichte der Dokumente.* [Based on the authors' study over six years of 5,000 pieces of archival material and on their identification of pertinent documents, mainly from the University of Vienna. Initially sponsored by the Sigmund Freud Archives, New York. Completed by Renée Gicklhorn after the death of Josef Gicklhorn in November 1957. With the text of forty documents and sample reproductions. With a bibliography.] Wien-Innsbruck, Urban & Schwarzenberg, 1960. 190 pp.

18. Ketchum, John Davidson. *Ruhleben; a prison camp society.* [An account of the social and psychological history of 4,000 British men and boys interned at Ruhleben, near Berlin, Germany, during the World War of 1914-1918. Based on the author's experience as a prisoner in Ruhleben, on contemporary and retrospective material he secured from 152 ex-prisoners, 1933-1961, including interviews in England and 116 questionnaires, and on the comprehensive collection of contemporary documents in the library of the Harvard University Law School.] With a foreword and postscript by Robert B. MacLeod. [With excerpts from contemporary diaries and letters mainly of thirteen prisoners. Completed by Robert B. MacLeod after the author's death in April 1962. With a bibliography of forty-nine books and articles dealing with Ruhleben, 1915-1938.] Toronto, Univ. of Toronto Pr.; London, Oxford Univ. Pr., 1965. 397 pp.

19. Evans, Richard Isadore. *Conversations with Carl Jung and reactions from Ernest Jones.* [Interviews with Jung filmed in Zurich in August 1957, and with Jones in Paris in July 1957 under the auspices of the Psychology Department of the University of Houston and the Radio

and Television Film Center at the University of Houston.] Princeton, N.J., London, Van Nostrand, 1964. 173 pp. (An Insight book, no. 23.)

20a. Ridenour, Nina A. *Mental health in the United States; a fifty-year history.* [Sponsored by the New York State Association for Mental Health.] Cambridge, Publ. for the Commonwealth Fund by Harvard Univ. Pr.; London, Oxford Univ. Pr., 1961. 146 pp.

20b. Montessori, Maria. *The Montessori method; scientific pedagogy as applied to child education in "the Children's Houses," with additions and revisions by the author* [transl. in part by Dorothy Canfield Fisher. Dedicated to the memory of Alice Hallgarten.] Transl. from the Italian [*Il metodo della pedagogica scientifica applicato all' educazione infantile nelle Case dei Bambini, Castello, 1909*] by Anne E. George. With an introd. by Martin Mayer. [Published originally in 1912, N.Y., Stokes. With publisher's foreword to the 1964 edition by Robert Bentley.] Cambridge, Mass., Bentley, 1964. 377 pp. Another ed.: *The Montessori method.* [Transl. by Anne E. George.] Introd. by J. McV. Hunt. [With a bibliography.] N.Y., Schocken Books, 1964. 376 pp. Paperback ed.: N.Y., Schocken Books, 1964. 376 pp. (SB88.)

20c. Montessori, Maria. *Dr. Montessori's own handbook.* [Authorized English translation, published originally in 1914, N.Y., Stokes; London, Heinemann.] Cambridge, Mass., Bentley, 1964, © 1914. 121 pp. Another ed.: Introd. by Nancy McCormick Rambush. N.Y., Schocken Books, 1965. 189 pp. Paperback ed.: N.Y. Schocken Books, 1965. 189 pp. (Schocken paperbacks, SB98.) Another ed. with title: *A Montessori handbook; "Dr. Montessori's own handbook."* Ed. by R. C. Orem, with additional new material on current Montessori theory and practice [by Genevieve Tarlton Alexander and others. With bibliographies.] N.Y., Putnam, 1966, © 1965. 192 pp. Paperback ed.: N.Y., Capricorn Books, Putnam, 1966, © 1965. 192 pp. (A Capricorn giant, 275.)

20d. Institute on Child Development in Kibbutzim, Oranim, Israel, etc., 1963. *Children in collectives; child-rearing aims and practices in the kibbutz.* [Proceedings of the one-week Institute, prepared under the auspices of Oranim, the Teachers' College in Israel, and the Child Development Center, New York. Participants: Moni Alon and others.] Ed. by Peter B. Neubauer. [Introd. by Gideon Lewin, Shimon Stern, and Nechama Levi. With five additional papers by Shmuel Golan and others. With a bibliography.] Springfield, Ill., Thomas, 1965. 383 pp.

20e. Rabin, Albert Israel. *Growing up in the kibbutz; comparison of the personality of children brought up in the kibbutz and of family-reared children.* [Based on the author's research with four age groups, one-year-old infants, ten-year-old children, seventeen-year-old adolescents, and nineteen- to twenty-year-old Army men, conducted in Israel in 1955 and 1962. With a bibliography.] N.Y., Springer, 1965. 230 pp.

20f. Spiro, Melford Elliot. *Children of the kibbutz.* [Based on the author's study during 1951-1952 of a kibbutz established thirty years previously.] With the assistance of Audrey G. Spiro. [Companion volume to the author's *Kibbutz; venture in utopia,* Cambridge, Mass., 1956; N.Y., 1963, © 1956.] Cambridge, Harvard Univ. Pr.; London, Oxford Univ. Pr., 1958. 500 pp. Paperback ed. with title: *Children of the kibbutz;* [a study in child training and personality. With a new pref. by the author.] N.Y., Schocken Books; London, Bailey & Swinfen [distributor], 1965. 500 pp. (Schocken paperbacks, SB93.)

21a. For example, studies of medicine and society in America, 1660-1860: Shryock, Richard Harrison. *Medicine and society in America, 1660-1860.* N.Y., New York Univ. Pr., 1960. 182 pp. (Anson G. Phelps lectureship on early American history, 1959.)

21b. the care of the insane, 1744-1845. Jones, Kathleen. *Lunacy, law and conscience, 1744-1845; the social history of the care of the insane.* N.Y., Grove Press; Humanities Press; London, Routledge & Paul, 1955. 239 pp. (International library of sociology and social reconstruction.)

21c. education and the handicapped, 1760-1960. Pritchard, David Gwyn. *Education and the handicapped, 1760-1960.* N.Y., Humanities Press [distributor] ; London, Routledge & Paul, 1963. 250 pp. (International library of sociology and social reconstruction.)

21d. mental health and social policy, 1845-1959. Jones, Kathleen. *Mental health and social policy, 1845-1959.* London, Routledge & Paul, 1960. 237 pp. (International library of sociology and social reconstruction.)

21e. immigrants and their children, 1850-1950. Hutchinson, Edward Prince. *Immigrants and their children, 1850-1950.* For the Social Science Research Council in cooperation with the U.S. Dept. of Commerce, Bureau of the Census. N.Y., Wiley; London, Chapman & Hall, 1956. 391 pp. (Census monograph series.)

22a. *See,* for example, three volumes in the series, "Perspectives in psychology," which present selected readings. Kessen, William, ed. *The child.* [Selected readings from modern Western sources, 1693-1942, with commentary. Series editors' foreword by George Mandler and William Kessen.] N.Y., London, Wiley, 1965. 301 pp. ("Perspectives in Psychology,") [covers 250 years, 1693-1942.]

22b. December, William Norton, ed. *Visual perception: the nineteenth century.* Selected readings with commentary. Series editors' foreword by George Mandler and William Kessen.] N.Y., London,

Wiley, 1964. 222 pp. ("Perspectives in psychology,") [covers the 19th century.]

22c. Anastasi, Anne, ed. *Individual differences.* [Excerpts from publications, 1869-1962, with commentary. Series editors' foreword by George Mandler and William Kessen.] N.Y., London, Wiley, 1965. 301 pp. ("Perspectives in psychology," covers the years 1869-1962.)

23. Harnack, Adolf von. "Bücher-Widmungen und Bücher-Titelaufnahmen: eine bibliographische Anregung." *Zentralblat für Bibliotheks-wesen,* 1924, 41, 177-182.

24. DeVore, Irven, ed. *Primate behavior: field studies of monkeys and apes.* [Outgrowth of a nine-month "Primate Project" and of two conferences held at the Center for Advanced Study in the Behavioral Sciences, Stanford, California, during 1962-1963. Organized by Sherwood L. Washburn and David A. Hamburg.] Contributors: Jarvis R. Bastian and others. [Dedicated to Clarence Ray Carpenter. With a bibliography.] N.Y., London, Holt, Rinehart & Winston, 1965. 654 pp.

25. Shor, Ronald Edwin, and Orne, Martin T., eds. *The nature of hypnosis; selected basic readings.* [Articles and excerpts from books and monographs previously published, 1784-1963. With bibliographies and an appendix: Selected bibliography on the history of hypnotism with primary emphasis on material available in the English language.] N.Y., London, Holt, Rinehart & Winston, 1965. 504 pp.

26. Boring, Edwin Garrigues. *History, psychology, and science; selected papers [1921-1963].* Ed. by Robert I. Watson and Donald T. Campbell. [With a bibliography.] N.Y., London, Wiley, 1963. 372 pp.

27. Lashley, Karl Spencer. *The neuropsychology of Lashley.* Ed. by Frank A. Beach, Donald O. Hebb, Clifford T. Morgan, and Henry W. Nissen. Introduction: Lashley and cortical integration, by Edwin G. Boring. A salute from neurologists, by Stabley Cobb. N.Y., London, McGraw-Hill, 1960. 564 pp. (McGraw-Hill series in psychology.)

28. Whorf, Benjamin Lee. *Language, thought, and reality.* Selected writings of Benjamin Lee Whorf. Ed. and with an introd. by John B. Carroll. Foreword by Stuart Chase. Cambridge, Mass., Technology Press of Massachusetts Institute of Technology; N.Y., Wiley; London, Chapman & Hall, 1956. 278 pp. (Technology Press books in the social sciences.)

29a. For examples *see:* Adler, Alfred. *Superiority and social interest: a collection of later writings* [1928-1937, transl. from the German, supplementing an earlier collection with title: *The individual psychology of Alfred Adler,* 1956.] Ed. by Heinz L. Ansbacher and Rowena R. Ansbacher. With a biographical essay by Carl Furtmüller. [With an exhaustive bibliography of the author's writings, 1898-1964.] Evanston, Ill., Northwestern Univ. Pr.; London, Routledge & Paul, 1964. 432 pp.

29b. Glueck, Sheldon, and Glueck, Eleanor. *Ventures in criminology; selected recent papers* [1953-1964. Dedicated to Hermann Mannheim and Benigno Di Tullio. With a chronological bibliography of the authors' publications, 1923-1963, initially compiled by Harvard Law School Library.] Cambridge, Harvard Univ. Pr., 1964. 373 pp. British ed.: Published under the auspices of the Institute for the Study and Treatment of Delinquency. London, Tavistock, 1964. 373 pp.

29c. Parsons, Talcott. *Social structure and personality.* [Eleven essays previously published, 1952-1961, and one previously unpublished essay. With a bibliography of the author's publications, 1928-1964.] N.Y., Free Press of Glencoe; London, Collier-Macmillan, 1964. 376 pp.

29d. Frederiksen, Norman, and Gulliksen, Harold, eds. *Contributions to mathematical psychology.* [Papers presented at a conference held by the Educational Testing Service in the spring of 1962 on the occasion of the dedication of a building in honor of Louis Leon Thurstone.] With chapters by Robert P. Abelson, Clyde H. Coombs, J. P. Guilford, Harold Gulliksen, Paul Horst, Ledyard R. Tucker, and Dorothy C. Adkins. [With a biographical paper and a complete bibliography of the published works of L. L. Thurstone, 1905-1959, by Dorothy C. Adkins.] N.Y., London, Holt, Rinehart & Winston, 1964. 189 pp.

29e. Gaskill, Herbert Stockton, ed. *Counterpoint; libidinal object and subject.* A tribute to René A. Spitz on his 75th birthday. [Papers and speeches of the celebration held under the auspices of the Department of Psychiatry, University of Colorado Medical Center, January 29, 1962. Participants: John D. Benjamin, Joan Fleming, Herbert S. Gaskill, Robert J. Glaser, Lawrence S. Kubie, Konrad Lorenz, Quigg Newton, Gerhart Piers, Leo Rangell, and René A. Spitz. With bibliographies and a list of publications by René A. Spitz, 1924-1963.] N.Y., International Universities Press, 1963. 200 pp.

29f. Grygier, Tadeusz, Jones, Howard, and Spencer, John Carrington, eds. *Criminology in transition; essays in honour of Hermann Mannheim* [to celebrate his seventy-fifth birthday. Series editors' foreword by Edward Glover and Emanuel Miller. With a biographical note by John Croft. With bibliographies and a bibliography of Mannheim's publications, 1912-1965. Published under the auspices of the Institute for the Study and Treatment of Delinquency.] South Hackensack, N.J., Rothman [distributor]; London, Tavistock, 1965. 308 pp. (International library of criminology, delinquency, and deviant social behaviour, no. 14.)

29g. Martin Scheerer Memorial Meetings on Cognitive Psychology, University of Kansas, 1962. *Cognition: theory, research, promise; papers, edited by Constance Scheerer.* [Contributors: Solomon E. Asch, John Ceraso, Riley W. Gardner, Fritz Heider, Sheldon J. Korchin, Joseph Lyons, C. Kermit Phelps, Irvin Rock, Ronald Taft, Seymour Wapner, and Herman A. Witkin. Under the editorship of Gardner Murphy. With bibliographies and a list of publications of Martin Scheerer, 1931-1961.] N.Y., London, Harper & Row, 1964. 226 pp.

29h. Waelder, Robert. *Psychoanalytic avenues to art.* [An expanded version of the lecture given at the New York Academy of Medicine on May 21, 1963. With a bibliography and a list of the author's publications, 1924-1965.] N.Y., International Universities Press, 1965. 122 pp. (The Freud anniversary lecture series of the New York Psychoanalytic Institute, 1963) London, Hogarth Press & Institute of Psycho-Analysis, 1965. 122 pp. (The Freud anniversary lecture series of the New York Psychoanalytic Institute, 1963. Psycho-analytical epitomes, no. 6.)

29i. Maier, Henry William. *Three theories of child development: the contributions of Erik H. Erikson, Jean Piaget, and Robert R. Sears, and their applications.* Under the editorship of [and with an introd. by] Werner W. Boehm. [Foreword by Dale B. Harris. With bibliographies and an appendix: The complete works of the three theorists: Erik H. Erikson: 1930-1964; Jean Piaget: 1924-1964; Robert R. Sears: 1936-1961.] N.Y., London, Harper & Row, 1965. 314 pp.

29j. Maslow, Abraham Harold. *Eupsychian management;* a journal [slightly edited from tape-recorded notes made by the author as invited Visiting Fellow at the Non-Linear Systems, Inc. plant in Del Mar, California, during the summer of 1962. Series editor's foreword by Warren G. Bennis. With a bibliography of the author's publications, 1932-1964.] Homewood, Ill., Irwin, 1965. 277 pp. (The Irwin-Dorsey series in behavioral science.)

30. Ilfeld, Fred, Jr., and Lauer, Roger. *Social nudism in America.* [A history, description, and analysis of the movement, based on the authors' field work in five southern California nudist camps during the summer of 1961 and on supplementary nudist literature. Outgrowth of a joint senior B.A. thesis in the honors program of Culture and Behavior and of Psychology of Yale University. With a bibliography.] New Haven, Conn., College and University Press, 1964. 240 pp. Paperback ed.: New Haven, Conn., College and University Press, 1964. 240 pp. (B-28.)

31. Menninger, Karl Augustus. *The vital balance; the life process in mental health and illness.* With Martin Mayman and Paul Pruyser. [With an appendix presenting a review of the psychiatric nosologies of all times.] N.Y., Viking Press, 1963. 531 pp.

32. Eissler, Kurt Robert. *Medical orthodoxy and the future of psychoanalysis.* [With an appendix: Challenges to Freud's honesty. A rebuttal of the Academic Lecture of 1956 by Percival Bailey: The great psychiatric revolution, *American Journal of Psychiatry,* 1956/57, 113, 387-406, and of Gicklhorn, J., and Gicklhorn, R., *Sigmund Freuds akademische Laufbahn im Lichte der Dokumente,* Wien, 1960. With a bibliography.] N.Y., International Universities Press, 1965. 592 pp.

33. Bayne, Helen, and Bry, Ilse. "Problems and Projects in the Bibliography of Psychiatry and Psychology." *Libri,* 1954, 3, 363-387. Bibliography: pp. 373-387.

34. Amacher, Peter. *Freud's neurological education and its influence on psychoanalytic theory.* [A study of pertinent neurological views of Freud's teachers, Ernst Brücke, Theodor Meynert, and Sigmund Exner, and their influence on Freud's views, traced through the beginnings of his psychoanalytic writings before 1900. Based on the author's doctoral dissertation in history, University of Washington, revised during a postdoctoral fellowship in the history of medicine at the University of California, Los Angeles, 1962-1964. With a bibliography.] N.Y., International Universities Press, 1965. 93 pp. (Psychological Issues, vol. 4, no. 4. Monograph 16.)

35. Schaller, George B. *The mountain gorilla; ecology and behavior.* [Report of the author's study as part of the African Primate Expedition, 1959-1961, under the direction of John T. Emlen, Jr. Based largely on direct observation during 314 encounters with gorillas. Dedicated to Olaus J. Murie. With a bibliography.] Chicago, London, Univ. of Chicago Pr., 1963. 431 pp.

36. Bullough, Vern Leroy. *The history of prostitution.* Bonnie L. Bullough, research associate. [With a bibliography and appendixes: I. Some English and American terms pertaining to prostitution from Chaucer to the present day. II. A bibliographic statement on the history of prostitution.] New Hyde Park, N.Y., University Books, 1964. 304 pp.

37. Farberow, Norman Louis, ed. *Taboo topics.* [Death, human sexual behavior, suicide, male homosexuality, parapsychology, graphology, religion, hypnosis, the psychologist in international affairs. Contributors: Daniel S. Anthony, William Douglas, Norman L. Farberow, Herman Feifel, Evelyn Hooker, Gardner Murphy, Charles E. Osgood, Wardell B. Pomeroy, Edwin S. Schneidman, and John G. Watkins. With selected bibliographies.] Foreword by Gordon W. Allport. N.Y., Atherton Press, 1963. 140 pp. (The Atherton Press behavioral science series) London, Prentice-Hall, 1963. 140 pp. (Behavioral Science series.)

38. 39. Bramson, Leon, and Goethals, George W., eds. *War: studies from psychology, sociology, anthropology.* [A collection of writings

previously published, 1863-1958. With a selected, classified bibliography.] N.Y., London, Basic Books, 1964. 407 pp.

40a. Group for the Advancement of Psychiatry. Committee on Mental Retardation. *Mental retardation: a family crisis—the therapeutic role of the physician.* Formulated by the Committee on Mental Retardation. [Dedicated to the memory of John Fitzgerald Kennedy. With appendixes: 1. Clinical entities. 2. Reading list for physicians. 3. Reading list for parents. Published in cooperation with the National Institute of Mental Health.] N.Y., Group for the Advancement of Psychiatry, 1963. pp. 116-148. (Group for the Advancement of Psychiatry. Report no. 56.)

40b. Osler, Sonia Fellner, and Cooke, Robert E., eds. *The biosocial basis of mental retardation.* [Lectures on the behavioral aspects of mental retardation presented in 1964 at the Johns Hopkins University School of Medicine. Contributors: Eli Ginzberg, Gary Griffin, Janet B. Hardy, Harry F. Harlow, Samuel A. Kirk, Austin Riesen, G. Wilson Shaffer, and David Zeaman. Dedicated to John F. Kennedy. With bibliographies.] Baltimore, Johns Hopkins Press, 1965; London, Oxford Univ. Pr., 1966. 151 pp.

40c. Fleishman, Edwin Alan. *The structure and measurement of physical fitness.* [Based on a project entitled *The Development of Criteria of Physical Fitness,* and on four progress reports of the research, including a nationwide study, carried out at Yale University, 1958-1962. A companion volume to the author's Examiner's manual for the basic fitness tests, Englewood Cliffs, N.J., 1964. Dedicated to John Fitzgerald Kennedy.] With a foreword by Stan Musial. [With a review of previous factor analysis studies in the area of physical fitness, catalogues of fitness and motor ability tests, and a bibliography.] Englewood Cliffs, N.J., London, Prentice-Hall, 1964. 207 pp.

40d. Abt, Lawrence Edwin, and Weissman, Stuart L., eds. *Acting out; theoretical and clinical aspects.* [A collection of invited papers with commentary. Dedicated to John Fitzgerald Kennedy. Foreword by Leopold Bellak. With case histories, reviews of the literature, and bibliographies.] N.Y., London, Grune & Stratton, 1965. 336 pp.

41. Bromberg, Walter. *Crime and the mind; a psychiatric analysis of crime and punishment.* [An enlargement and revision of the author's *Crime and the mind; an outline of psychiatric criminology,* Philadelphia, 1948. With case material, including a case history of Jack Ruby. With bibliographies.] N.Y., Macmillan; London, Collier-Macmillan, 1965. 431 pp.

42. Wolfenstein, Martha, and Kliman, Gilbert, eds. *Children and the death of a President; multi-disciplinary studies* [discussed in pre-

liminary form as work in progress at a conference on "Children's Reactions to the Death of the President," held in April 1964 at the Albert Einstein College of Medicine. Contributors: Augusta Alpert and others. Pref. by Joseph B. Cramer. With case examples and bibliographies. With appendixes: Essays of junior high school students in a suburb of New York, written January 29, 1964, on: "What I remember about the weekend when President Kennedy was assassinated," and Transcript of tape-recorded interviews by Dr. Kliman with children ages seven to twelve, in a suburb of New York, November 23-25, 1963.] Garden City, N.Y., Doubleday, 1965. 256 pp. Paperback ed.: Garden City, N.Y., Anchor Books, Doubleday, 1966. 288 pp. (A Doubleday anchor book, A543.)

# ESSAY 11

## *"Intensive Bibliography" and the Growth Pattern of the Literature in the Behavioral Sciences*

Originally published as Editorial in *Mental Health Book Review Index*, vol. 14 (whole no. 19), 1969.

### GROWTH IN AN EXTENSIVE AND INTENSIVE DIMENSION

Scientific literature grows in more than one dimension. Its extensive growth, the increase in the sheer number of publications, has become explosive in our time but was deplored in surprisingly similar terms in previous generations. Its growth in the intensive dimension, the gain in substance which reflects the progress of knowledge, has not been so readily apparent. In science relatively few contributions are recognized as classic and stay alive in their original form. Many more are transformed and absorbed. An indefinite number of scientific writings that are added to the literature do not contribute to knowledge and leave no trace in the more stringent records of the advancement of science. Usually, the terms "growth," "growth rate," or "growth pattern" of scientific literature refer only to estimates of the quantity of certain types of publications, e.g., journals, journal articles, abstracts, and so forth, which appeared in print at various times. If, however, qualitative factors such as significance, validity, impact, and durability were taken into consideration, in other words, if the basic concept would encompass both the intensive and extensive dimension, the growth of scientific literature would show the pattern of a pyramid, which narrows as it rises from its base.

This pattern prevails in many cultural processes that begin with a mass of individual components and end with selective representation. The same principle is applied in sampling, from wine tasting through opinion polls to controlled research studies. Applied to scientific literature, the principle of selective representation would lead us to ask, not how much has been published, but how little of that do we need in order to keep a meaningful record of scientific progress? The pursuit of this question suggests "intensive bibliography" as a new concept and approach.

## PERPLEXITIES OF THE PAST

Although scientists have not yet dealt in a scientific way with the intensive growth of their literature, they have considered it in theory and contributed to it in practice. From time to time, the challenge of expansion at the base has been met by new ideas for contraction. The Chinese, who began in the sixth century to compile encyclopedias, are credited with having invented them in their desire to bring together condensed, yet precise, information about a large variety of subjects. The rise of scientific journals, the first of which appeared in France in 1665, has been attributed to the need of the mercantile system for knowledge about foreign developments in science. The first journals consisted of extracts from books, then the only form of primary publication. They are, therefore, the forerunner of scientific journals, book reviews, abstracts, and abstracting and information services.

The various forms of condensation have often changed in both nature and name. To define them requires a historical orientation, for which a firm basis is lacking. An encyclopedia, for example, is supposed to summarize, in Diderot's words, "the knowledge scattered over the surface of the earth." The largest of all encyclopedias, however, the *Yung Lo Ta Tien,* compiled early in the 15th century in 22,937 books, was neither universal nor concise. Since the 19th century, encyclopedias confined to a branch of knowledge have outnumbered those that still try to be all-embracing. Subject encyclopedias may also be called *Handbuch* or "handbook," a name used for desk manuals as well as for monumental systematizations of knowledge; their title, such as *Psychology: a Study of a Science* (6 vols., 1959-1963), may not even show their encyclopedic ancestry and nature. Thus, works that appear similar in name or format may actually differ greatly—or vice versa—depending on the tradition they follow and the function they fulfill.

This applies also to other familiar forms, especially to abstracts. In the 18th century, extracts from books, periodicals, and dissertations were up to ten or even more pages long and gave a report of contents without criticism. This changed in the 19th century, when the German *Zentralblätter* and similar abstracting journals met the growing need for selection and evaluation. Besides critical abstracts of books and journal articles there were scientific book reviews which followed the tradition of the humanities. The trend has been for book reviews to remain evaluative—supplemented by shorter book notes—for abstracts, to become briefer, noncritical, and limited to the journal literature. However, a noncritical abstracting journal such as *Psychological Abstracts* may also include books.

The tendency of abstracting journals to become less and less selective has repeatedly caused great concern. It raises the problem that, when they cannot really be comprehensive, they may omit material on practical rather than reject it on scholarly grounds. The value of using authors' abstracts, once the exception and now increasingly the rule, has also long been debated. In a scholarly abstracting journal, editors and contributors add their own competence in selecting an article for abstracting and bringing out its essence. To reprint routinely the authors' abstracts that have become a required adjunct to the original article is no substitute because it omits this added intellectual process.

## THE COMPUTER AT THE CROSSROADS

In the hope for greater speed and future savings, the step from authors' abstracts to auto-abstracting through a mechanical process by computer was first attempted in the 1950's. Efforts to find a basis for programming a computer have led to research into various aspects of the problem, ranging from a study of abstracters' instructions and criteria for acceptable abstracts (H. Borko and S. Chatman, *American*

*Documentation,* April 1963) to studies of the underlying processes of human communication.

In using computers for bibliographic purposes, comparable research will have to be developed. The prevailing one-sided use of computers has had a depressant effect on the growth pattern of scientific literature: it reflects the inflated extensive growth and obscures, if it does not actually inhibit, the growth in the intensive dimension. In order to achieve a better balance, studies are needed which would analyze the criteria and processes involved in bibliographic selection.

For example, scientific bibliographic services have traditionally been concerned with "primary" publications, mainly the journal literature and other material containing new data and information. These services themselves are "secondary" publications, a term that applies to all types of publications which index, abstract, and review the primary literature or compile data from it. This distinction has had consequences for the bibliographic system as a whole. It is well known that not every "primary" publication is also original and a contribution. Those that are not are included in so many indexing and abstracting services because of the cost and problems of making a selection. On the other hand, "secondary" publications that are critical and selective, especially the annual reviews and topical review articles, can be original in thought–for example, by offering a new conceptual integration–and can contribute to knowledge by helping to establish it.

The place of these secondary publications in the literature is not clear. In the scientific community, attitudes toward them are conflicting and ambivalent. Good critical reviews, which require exceptional competence and breadth of vision, are highly respected. Many scientific journals publish, however, only reports of primary research or articles not available in other sources. The growing literature directly concerned with the review of scientific progress has been isolated. It appears in the form of serials, occasional articles, and separate books. The bibliographic treatment which these "secondary" publications receive is uncertain, incomplete, and usually incidental. In particular, few attempts have been made to use them as sources for further, specific bibliographic treatment, aimed at an already sifted and integrated scientific literature. In principle, the citation indexes have been a move in this direction; yet their present magnitude and complexity appears to obscure their full potential. Perhaps their inventors have not gone far enough in developing this 20th-century innovation.

The general trend in using computers in science information has, therefore, been to keep bibliographic processes close to the base of the pyramid, even those that used to be carried out on a higher level. It is here proposed to do the opposite: to direct bibliographic effort to the upper levels of the pyramid, where knowledge can be found in a more concentrated state. The processes or works that contribute to the goal of achieving a concentration of knowledge may be called "intensifiers," at least until a better name may be found. The term should suggest an advanced level of scholarship, not a secondary pursuit in science. The new type of bibliography would take the "intensifiers" as its starting point and incorporate them and their results into the bibliographic record. This approach is here called "intensive bibliography." When it has been developed, it will have access to intellectually powerful data, which will make the use of computers more challenging and productive.

## THE INTENSIFIERS IN PRINCIPLE

The following analysis suggests objectives and processes which play a part in the intensive growth of scientific literature.

The oldest and still the highest aim is to provide *synthesis and direction,* which is the *encyclopedic* function. In the eyes of the Encyclopedists and their intellectual heirs in the 20th century, an encyclopedia should seek to "make comprehensible," not to "make known." Daring and *avant-garde,* it should hope "to change the world for the better" and be "an invitation to the present generation to examine its intellectual conscience"—not recent ideas, but still fit to serve as a model and criterion for the current encyclopedias in the social and behavioral sciences. *Selection and coordination* are the most immediate task in *surveying* the progress made during a limited period, often the preceding year. Under various names, the "progress series" and other types of topical reviews discuss the development of a field or problem, point out the significance of new findings and trends, give recognition to the contributing scientists, and cite the important, critically selected literature.

Review articles and essay reviews, which discuss a group of books on a given subject, form a transition from the topical review of progress to the evaluation of a single book. *Assessment and accentuation* of the significance of a book in comparison with related works are expected from the scientific *book review* in any form. With the increase and scattering of journal articles, *synopsis and information* have become the main function of *abstracts*, on the assumption that their users "want meat without parsley or trimmings" (E. J. Crane, *Special Libraries*, July-August 1940).

The intellectual requirements of *analysis and reorganization* make *indexing* more difficult than abstracting. Subject indexing, especially, calls for an adequate understanding of the particular subject matter and a general knowledge of the field. Without anticipating the later indexes of keywords used in titles, which involve the authors' cooperation as well as the aid of computers, Crane (*ibid.*) cautioned against indexing that was too much guided by titles. *Citation and organization* are the elements of *bibliography*, not in the sense that they are simple but because they are fundamental. The bibliographic function, which enters into every kind of work with scientific literature, is the most flexible of all. Contributions in bibliographic form range from footnotes that document specific statements to exhaustive, classified, and annotated subject bibliographies. It is noteworthy that this instrument of scientific literature has been both base and target of intensive bibliography, first in the form of bibliographies of bibliography, more recently through the bibliographic re-use of citations.

By serving the need for *retrospection and reintegration*, the vertically oriented *cumulation* complements the horizontally oriented review of recent advances. In the history of scientific literature, cumulation has played a now rather forgotten role, beginning with collections of various kinds in the 17th century and continuing with cumulative indexes to journals in the 18th century. Both have their counterparts today. Significantly, within the past year, three journals in our field, *Social Service Review*, *Eugenics Review*, and *Psychiatry*, have issued cumulative indexes, covering, respectively, 40, 60, and 30 years, with the aim, as stated by the Editor of *Psychiatry*, of ensuring "that ideas will remain alive as seminal agents in the cumulative growth of shared knowledge."

Most unstructured and unpredictable are the intensifiers that perform an immediate scholarly service through *comment* and *correction*, often concerned with a specific point. They cannot be identified with any single literary form. The more typical forms are the *discussions* that are a part of the proceedings of scientific meetings; the *letter to the editor;* the *rejoinder;* the *correction* and *erratum;* and the *editorial com-*

*ment* or *note.* Perhaps the most enigmatic literary form in science, the *editorial,* should be included here. It is being used in as many ways as editors of scientific journals choose. When it anticipates major problems and guides opinion toward their attack and solution, it fulfills, in the fragmentized world of modern specialization, a function of the great encyclopedias, and so closes the circle.

The literary forms and functions that are here linked with specific objectives are not limited to them. Each of these forms may serve its own immediate purpose best when it also fulfills as many of the other objectives as it can reasonably encompass. For example, a bibliography must cite and organize, but it makes a greater contribution when it also selects and coordinates, as does the literature survey, and provides synthesis and direction, as does the encyclopedia. The forms or functions are, therefore, not "intensifiers" because they have a certain format or follow a certain technique. Rather, they become "intensifiers" when, and only when, they help achieve a given objective.

## A BEGINNING OF INTENSIVE BIBLIOGRAPHY IN THE BEHAVIORAL SCIENCES

The behavioral sciences, perhaps making a virtue of necessity, have long been cultivating the intensive growth of their literature. Seemingly late in adopting the intensifying devices of the 19th century, they are now leading in developing their own. They have loosened the rigid structure of traditional channels and adapted or created functional literary forms. The behavioral sciences have no counterpart in other areas of science in wealth of monographic literature and in cross-disciplinary communication through book reviews. This book-review literature is, therefore, a natural starting ground for intensive bibliography. The *Mental Health Book Review Index* has used it as a basis for pursuing the idea of selective representation, as the following examples may illustrate.

As a result of the critical judgments made by the specialists who select books for review, a large proportion of the books listed in the *Index* represent themselves work on the higher levels of the pyramid. These include handbooks in special fields[1,2]; surveys of theories that have been of consequence in the behavioral sciences[3]; and reviews of the research literature. In the current volume, literature surveys cover research in psychology[4]; meaning[5]; positive mental health[6]; child development[7]; childbearing from a social-science viewpoint[8]; schizophrenia and the poor[9]; drug addiction[10,11]; and drug therapy.[12] In addition, extensive reviews of research appear in books on various subjects, e.g., depression[13]; stuttering[14]; underachievers[15]; and violence.[16] Historical surveys of concepts such as intelligence, alienation, and identity[17,18,19] complement the reviews of "antecedent research."[20,21,22] The *Index* entries identify these books as sources of such topical reviews, even if the titles do not. The method that is basic to the *Index*–listing books with the references to groups of multidisciplinary reviews and repeating these listings when more multiple reviews can be cited–has become an intensifying device. When the time span of book reviews is extended over many years, or when work done many decades ago is still being reevaluated, the book reviews may help to answer the question: "What is a classic in the behavioral sciences?"[23,24,25,26,27]

Review articles and essay reviews are cited with their titles. These range from a critical notice (the British name for thorough evaluations of significant books) from the U.S.S.R. by A. R. Luria, who reviews an international symposium on brain and conscious experience held in Rome,[28] and another critical notice of one of the reviewer's books on higher nervous activity in man,[29] to a psychoanalytic review of twelve books on parapsychology[30,31]; from annual reviews of books in pastoral psychology[32] to periodic surveys of paperbacks in psychology.[33] A cross between book reviews and other literary forms is suggested in such variants as "an editorial review"[34] and, "Three book reviews: a memorial to David Rapaport."[35] The growing number of essay reviews in the area of social issues focuses on urban problems[36,37,38]; race relations; Negro life[39,40]; poverty[41,42,43,44]; and deviance and the disadvantaged.[45,46] These review articles highlight the interlocking of many of these problems, as different reviewers may discuss the same books in one or another context. The function of literature surveys to point out significant trends is very evident here; so is the fact that much of this research and its critical discussion antedates, often by many years, the more recent public awareness.

Works that serve the reintegration of the past with the present in the form of collections, complete authors' bibliographies, dedications, and other contributions to the history of ideas were discussed in the editorial in Volume 12, 1967, of the *Index*. The corresponding bibliographic techniques are, therefore, not mentioned here again. More bibliographic innovations are needed, however, in order to derive the full benefit from the last group of intensifiers described earlier. The *Index* includes book reviews that are published as editorials and cites comments and corrections together with the original reference, whether or not they appear together in the journals indexed. They are usually critical comments made by authors or others on the review, often followed by the reviewer's reply, or corrections made by the editor, a reader, or the reviewer himself.

In rarer yet significant instances, the scope of these communications broadens the dialogue and their message is of general interest. For example, a group of letters, one of them signed by 23 well-known British psychiatrists, while written to protest the tenor of a book review, actually greatly enhance the tribute to Sir Aubrey Lewis intended by his students who issued two volumes of his selected writings.[47,48] The elements of a ghost reference that attributes to Gertrude Stein a paper on the effect of repetition on memory in the *Psychological Review* of 1896, are disentangled in a comment on a review of the recent biography of William James by Gay Wilson Allen.[49] Another attempt to dissolve a legend before it can take hold in the literature of the behavioral sciences is made by Heinz L. Ansbacher. He points out that the designation of Freud as chairman of the 1910 discussion on suicide in the recently published English translation is neither authentic with respect to the German original nor true with respect to the facts, an emendation then confirmed by the editor of the book.[50] There is at present no established procedure for incorporating such corrections into the bibliographic entries. It would be important, however, to design methods of fully integrating later corrections with the previous scientific and bibliographic information, especially when this is stored in a computer. This problem should have a high priority in developing intensive bibliography.

The *Cumulative Author-Title Index, Volumes 1-12, 1956-1967,* applies for the first time the intensifying force of a cumulative index to the book-review literature encompassed by the *Mental Health Book Review Index* during that period. This leads to a high degree of concentration. Within less than 200 pages, brief bibliographic citations, supplemented by a host of cross references, will provide a key to the nearly 4,000 books listed in the *Index* up to 1967. Many of these review the literature of their respective subjects or present a new synthesis of knowledge in another form, and they, in turn, have been evaluated in the book reviews—totaling more than 22,000—which are cited in the first twelve volumes of the *Index*.

Further studies should be facilitated and, it is hoped, encouraged by this cumulative index. They might show to what extent the *Index* is achieving its aim to develop a body of literature that is a representative sample rather than an aggregate of current monographic publications relating to the behavioral sciences. This would mean that eminent and still influential authors of the formative periods and those who have made significant contemporary contributions should have a place in this list; that the important topics and trends which have engaged the special attention of the scientific community in the behavioral sciences since the mid-1950's should become apparent; and that the field as a whole, which has no structural boundaries, should be delineated in a dynamic synthesis of progress. In short, the cumulative index should help to put to a test the potential of this pioneer effort to make intensive bibliography itself an intensifier that can span the entire range of objectives, from the encyclopedic to the corrective functions.

## REFERENCES AND NOTES

1. Gordon, Jesse Emanuel, ed. *Handbook of clinical and experimental hypnosis.* [Contributors: Frank A. Pattie and others. With case illustrations, reviews of the literature, and bibliographies.] N.Y., Macmillan; London, Collier-Macmillan, 1967. 653 pp.

2. Magary, James F., ed. *School psychological services in theory and practice; a handbook.* [Chapters by Robert M. Allen and others on developments since the publication of the Thayer Conference on the Functions, Qualifications, and Training of School Psychologists, West Point, N.Y., 1954, School psychologists at mid-century, Washington, 1955. With reviews of the literature and bibliographies.] Englewood Cliffs, N.J., Prentice-Hall, 1967. 774 pp. (Prentice-Hall psychology series.)

3. Baldwin, Alfred Lee. *Theories of child development.* [Dedicated to the memory of Gordon S. Ieradi. With a bibliography.] N.Y., London, Wiley, 1966, © 1967. 618 pp.

4. *Annual review of psychology.* Vol. 18, 1967. Paul R. Farns-

worth, editor; Olga McNemar, associate editor; Quinn McNemar, associate editor. [Editorial Committee (1967): G. W. Albee and others. Responsible for organization of vol. 18: E. S. Bordin, K. E. Clark, L. J. Cronbach, P. R. Farnsworth, F. A. Geldard, and H. H. Kelley. With bibliographies.] Palo Alto, Calif., Annual Reviews, 1967. 606 pp.

5. Creelman, Marjorie Broer. *The experimental investigation of meaning; a review of the literature.* [With bibliographies.] N.Y., Springer, 1966. 228 pp.

6. Davis, James Allan. *Education for positive mental health; a review of existing research and recommendations for future studies* [undertaken to answer questions raised at the National Assembly on Mental Health Education, 1958, sponsored by Pennsylvania Mental Health, Inc., and others. Pref. by Norman M. Bradburn. With a bibliography including an annotated bibliography of experimental studies.] Chicago, Aldine, 1965. 192 pp. (National Opinion Research Center. Monographs in social research, 5.)

7. Hoffman, Lois Norma Wladis, and Hoffman, Martin Leon, eds. *Review of child development research.* Vol. 2. [By Henry Borow and others.] Prepared under the auspices of the Society for Research in Child Development. [Advisory Committee: Nancy Bayley and others. Editorial consultants: Aline B. Auerbach and others. With bibliographies.] N.Y., Russell Sage Foundation, 1966. 598 pp. (Publications of Russell Sage Foundation.)

8. Richardson, Stephen Alexander, and Guttmacher, Alan Frank, eds. *Childbearing: its social and psychological aspects.* [A series of critical reviews, by Elaine R. Grimm, Ernest M. Gruenberg, Raymond Illsley, Margaret Mead, Niles Newton, and Jay S. Rosenblatt, of studies of reproduction oriented toward a social-science viewpoint. Outgrowth of a recommendation of the Perinatal Research Committee, established by the National Institute of Neurological Diseases and Blindness. Published under the auspices of the Association for the Aid of Crippled Children. With bibliographies.] Baltimore, Williams & Wilkins; Edinburgh, Livingstone [distributor], 1967. 334 pp.

9. Roman, Paul M., and Trice, Harrison Miller. *Schizophrenia and the poor.* [An evaluation of research studies and a review of the literature on mental disorder and social status. With bibliographies.] Ithaca, New York State School of Industrial and Labor Relations, Cornell University, 1967. 78 pp. (ILR paperback no. 3.)

10. Kalant, Oriana Josseau. *The amphetamines; toxicity and addiction.* [A survey of the literature undertaken at the request of the Department of Health of the Government of Ontario. Foreword by E. A. Sellers. With case histories and a bibliography.] Springfield, Ill.,

Thomas, 1966. 151 pp. (Brookside monographs, no. 5.)

11. Silberman, Martin. *Aspects of drug addiction; a report on a survey carried out under the auspices of the Royal London Prisoners' Aid Society.* [A review of the literature, with comments based on interviews with physicians, social workers, and drug users. Prefatory statement by A. M. G. Christopher. Foreword by Thomas H. Bewley.] London, Royal London Prisoners' Aid Society, 1967. 112 pp.

12. Wittenborn, John Richard. *The clinical psychopharmacology of anxiety.* [A review and assessment of the reports of controlled studies of pharmacotherapies used in the management of anxiety in non-schizophrenic patients, 1960-1965. With a report of the author's analysis of combined data provided by Wyeth Laboratories and in a collaborative study with the New Jersey State Department of Institutions and Agencies by the author and his associates, 1963-1964. With a bibliography.] Springfield, Ill., Thomas, 1966. 228 pp.

13. Beck, Aaron Temkin. *Depression: clinical, experimental, and theoretical aspects.* [Based in part on a five-year research project with more than 1,000 patients conducted by the author with K. Erbaugh and others at the University of Pennsylvania and on data collected in the course of the psychotherapy of depressed patients. With an appendix: Depression inventory. With extensive reviews of the literature and a bibliography.] N.Y., London, Hoeber Medical Division, Harper & Row, 1967. 370 pp.

14. Freund, Henry. *Psychopathology and the problems of stuttering, with special consideration of clinical and historical aspects.* [Outgrowth of the author's personal experience, his clinical work with stuttering school children and adults as chief of several speech clinics and in private practice of logopedics in Yugoslavia, 1932-1940, and of his work for 25 years as a psychiatrist in the United States. Based in part on the author's publications in European and American journals.] With a foreword by Charles Van Riper. [With extensive reviews of the literature and a bibliography.] Springfield, Ill., Thomas, 1966. 233 pp. (American lecture series, publ. no. 641. American lectures in speech and hearing.)

15. Raph, Jane Beasley, Goldberg, Miriam L., and Passow, A. Harry. *Bright underachievers; studies of scholastic underachievement among intellectually superior high school students.* [Based on two studies conducted by the Talented Youth Project at the Evanston Township High School, Evanston, Illinois, 1955-1956, and on three studies conducted at De Witt Clinton High School, Bronx, New York, 1956-1961. Foreword by Arthur W. Foshay. With excerpts from interview data. With a comprehensive review of the literature and a bibliography. Pub-

lished for the Horace Mann-Lincoln Institute of School Experimentation, Talented Youth Project.] N.Y., Teachers College Press, 1966. 289 pp.

16. Wolfgang, Marvin Eugene, and Ferracuti, Franco. *The subculture of violence; towards an integrated theory in criminology.* [Translated from the Italian, *Il comportamento violento: moderni aspetti criminologici,* Milano, 1966. Dedicated to Thorsten Sellin and Benigno Di Tullio. Foreword by Hermann Mannheim. With extensive reviews of the literature and bibliographies.] N.Y., Barnes & Noble [distributor]; London, Tavistock, 1967. 387 pp. Paperback ed.: N.Y., Barnes & Noble [distributor]; London, Tavistock, 1967. 387 pp. (Social science paperbacks, 16.)

17. Guilford, Joy Paul. *The nature of human intelligence.* [With a historical survey of tests and concepts of intelligence. With reviews of the literature and an extensive bibliography.] N.Y., London, McGraw-Hill, 1967. 538 pp. (McGraw-Hill series in psychology.)

18. Hammond, Guyton Bowers. *Man in estrangement; a comparison of the thought of Paul. Tillich and Erich Fromm.* [Foreword by Langdon Gilkey. With a review of the concept of estrangement (alienation) and a bibliography.] Nashville, Vanderbilt Univ. Pr., London, C. Hurst [distributor], 1965. 194 pp.

19. Levita, David Joël de. *The concept of identity.* With a pref. by H. C. Rümke. [Translated by Ian Finlay. With reviews of the literature, a summary in English and Dutch, and bibliographies. Issued also as thesis, University of Utrecht.] The Hague, Mouton, 1965; N.Y., Basic Books, 1967, © 1965. 209 pp. (New Babylon; studies in the behavioral sciences, 2.)

20. Hartmann, Ernest. *The biology of dreaming.* [Based in part on the author's research. Subseries editor's foreword by I. Newton Kugelmass. With reviews of pertinent studies and a bibliography.] Springfield, Ill., Thomas, 1967, 206 pp. (Boston State Hospital monograph series, no. 2.) (American lecture series, publ. no. 686. American lectures in living chemistry.)

21. Pasamanick, Benjamin, Scarpitti, Frank R., and Denitz, Simon. *Schizophrenics in the community; an experimental study in the prevention of hospitalization* [designed in 1957 at the Psychiatric Institute and Hospital, Department of Psychiatry, Ohio State University in cooperation with the Research Division of the Columbus Psychiatric Institute and Hospital and carried out, beginning in 1961, with 152 state hospital schizophrenic patients and 52 ambulatory schizophrenic patients at the Institute Treatment Center, Louisville, Kentucky]. With the collaboration of Joseph Albini and Mark Lefton. [Foreword by Stanley

F. Yolles. With a review of antecedent research and case history documents.] N.Y., Appleton-Century-Crofts, 1967. 448 pp. (Sociology series.)

22. Stone, Philip J., Dunphy, Dexter C., Smith, Marshall S., and Ogilvie, Daniel M. *The general inquirer; a computer approach to content analysis.* [Report of research conducted since 1961 under the auspices of the Laboratory of Social Relations, Harvard University.] With associates [and contributors: Ole R. Holsti and others. Dedicated to Robert F. Bales. Foreword by Harold Lasswell. With a historical review of content analysis research. With bibliographies.] Cambridge, Mass., M.I.T. Press, 1966. 651 pp.

23. American Journal of Orthopsychiatry. *Child guidance: Lawson G. Lowrey memorial volume.* Edited [with a biographical sketch: Lawson G. Lowrey, M.D., 1890-1957, and a summary of the papers given at the Lawson G. Lowrey memorial meeting held in New York City, March 7, 1958] by Simon H. Tulchin. A collection of papers which appeared in the *American Journal of Orthopsychiatry* during the years of 1930 through 1957. Editorial Committee: David M. Levy, Frederika Neumann, and Simon H. Tulchin, chairman. [Contributors: Smith Ely Jeliffe and others. With case material and excerpts from discussions. With a list of Lowrey's publications, 1911-1957. With bibliographies.] N.Y., American Orthopsychiatric Association, 1964. 380 pp.

24. Craik, Kenneth James Williams. *The nature of psychology; a selection of papers, essays, and other writings.* Edited by Stephen L. Sherwood. [Introd. by Warren S. McCulloch, Leo Verbeek, and Stephen L. Sherwood. With an obituary notice: Kenneth J. W. Craik, 1914-1945, by F. C. Bartlett, reprinted from the *British Journal of Psychology,* General Section, 1946, 36, 109. With a list of the author's publications, 1937-1948, compiled by Mrs. S. J. Macpherson. With a bibliography.] N.Y., London, Cambridge Univ. Pr., 1966. 184 pp.

25. Friedman, Paul, ed. *On suicide, with particular reference to suicide among young students.* Discussions of the Vienna Psychoanalytic Society–1910. With contributions by Alfred Adler, Sigmund Freud [chairman], Josef K. Friedjung, Karl Molitor, David Ernst Oppenheim, Rudolf Reitler, J. [Isidor] Sadger, and Wilhelm Stekel. [Translated from the German, Wiener Psychoanalytische Vereinigung, Über den Selbstmord, Wien, 1910, as a project of the Library Committee of the New York Psychoanalytic Institute. Translation first drafted by Edward Fitzgerald.] Edited [and with a historical review of the literature] by Paul Friedman. [Pref. by Alfred Adler. With case material.] N.Y., International Universities Press; London, Bailey & Swinfen [distributor], 1967. 121 pp.

26. Horney, Karen. *Feminine psychology.* [Ten papers previously published, 1924-1935, and five papers previously published in German, 1926/27-1937, reprinted in translation by Edward C. Clemmens, John M. Meth, Edward Schattner, and Gerda F. Willner, Editorial Committee.] Edited and with an introd. by Harold Kelman, [chairman, Editorial Committee. Sponsored by the Association for the Advancement of Psychoanalysis.] N.Y., Norton, 1967. 269 pp. London, Routledge & Paul, 1967. 271 pp.

27. Lewin, Louis. *Phantastica; narcotic and stimulating drugs, their use and abuse.* [Reprinted from the first English ed., London, 1931, with a new] foreword by Bo Holmstedt. [Translated from the 2nd German ed., *Phantastica; die betäubenden und erregenden Genussmittel,* Berlin, 1927, by P. H. A. Wirth. With case illustrations.] N.Y., Dutton; London, Routledge & Paul, 1964. 335 pp.

28. Pontificia Accademia delle Scienze, Rome. *Brain and conscious experience.* Study Week, September 28 to October 4, 1964, of the Pontificia Academia Scientiarum; [papers and discussions. Participants: Lord Adrian of Cambridge and others.] Edited by John C. Eccles. [Dedicated to the memory of C. S. Sherrington and E. Schrödinger. Originally published in volume 30 of *Pontificiae Academiae Scientiarum Scripta Varia.*] N.Y., Springer, 1966, © 1965. 591 pp.

29. Luriia, Aleksandr Romanovich. *Human brain and psychological processes, by A. R. Luria.* 1966. [Based on a series of studies carried out between 1938 and 1963 in the Institute of Neurology and the N. N. Burdenko Institute of Neurosurgery of the USSR Academy of Medical Sciences. Ten papers, mostly previously unpublished, written or revised in 1962.] Translated [from the Russian *Mozg cheloveka i psikhicheskie protsessy,* Moscow, 1963] by Basil Haigh. [Under the editorship of Gardner Murphy and Wayne Holtzman. Prefaces by Hans-Lukas Teuber and Karl H. Pribram. With case reports and a bibliography.] N.Y., London, Harper & Row, 1966. 587 pp.

30. Eisenbud, Jule. *The world of Ted Serios; "thoughtographic" studies of an extraordinary mind.* [With illustrated examples and a bibliography.] N.Y., Morrow, 1967; London, Cape, 1968. 367 pp.

31. Thouless, Robert Henry. *Experimental psychical research.* [Editorial foreword by C. A. Mace. With reviews of the literature and a bibliography.] Harmondsworth, Middlesex, Penguin Books, 1963; Baltimore, Penguin Books, 1964, © 1963. 148 pp. (Pelican books, A623; a Pelican original.)

32. Rogers, Carl Ransom, ed. *The therapeutic relationship and its impact; a study of psychotherapy with schizophrenics.* [Report of a research program conducted by the Psychotherapy Research Group,

University of Wisconsin Psychiatric Institute, with the cooperation of Mendota State Hospital. Authors: Carl R. Rogers, Eugene T. Gendlin, Donald J. Kiesler, Charles B. Truax, Philippa L. Mathieu, and Marjorie H. Klein. Contributing authors: Byron L. Barrington and others. Commentators: Paul Bergman and others.] Edited by Carl R. Rogers with the collaboration of Eugene T. Gendlin, Donald J. Kiesler, and Charles B. Truax. [With excerpts from therapy samples and bibliographies.] Madison, London, Univ. of Wisconsin Pr., 1967. 625 pp.

33. Matson, Floyd W. *The broken image; man, science and society.* [With a bibliography.] N.Y. Braziller, 1964. 355 pp. Paperback ed.: Garden City, N.Y., Anchor Books, Doubleday, 1966. 342 pp. (A Doubleday anchor book, A506.)

34. Delacato, Carl Henry. *Neurological organization and reading.* [With the edited reports of ten studies by Roxana Carrick and others, concerned with the scientific appraisal of the concept of neurological organization as applied to the diagnosis and treatment of reading problems.] Springfield, Thomas, 1966. 189 pp.

35. Holt, Robert Rutherford, ed. *Motives and thought: psychoanalytic essays in honor of David Rapaport,* [by Benjamin B. Rubinstein, George S. Klein, Roy Schafer, Lester Luborsky, I. H. Paul, Merton M. Gill, Peter H. Wolff, and Robert R. Holt]. Edited [and with an introductory essay: David Rapaport: a memoir (September 30, 1911-December 14, 1960)] by Robert R. Holt. [With a bibliography.] N.Y., International Universities Press, 1967. 413 pp. (Psychological Issues, vol. 5, no. 2-3. Monograph 18/19.)

36. Banton, Michael Parker. *The policeman in the community.* [Based on research started in 1960 in Scotland and on comparative inquiries in the United States and Sweden, 1961-1963.] N.Y., Basic Books; London, Tavistock, 1964. 276 pp.

37. Hauser, Philip Morris, and Schnore, Leo Francis, eds. *The study of urbanization.* [Based on the proceedings of the Committee on Urbanization, Social Science Research Council, 1958-1964, Philip M. Hauser, chairman. Contributors: Norton S. Ginsburg and others. With a historical bibliographical survey by Charles N. Glaab and two other supplementary papers by Harold M. Mayer and Brian J. L. Berry. With bibliographies.] N.Y., London, Wiley, 1965. 554 pp.

38. Stahl, David, Sussman, Frederick B., and Bloomfield, Neil J., eds. *The community and racial crises.* [Based on a three-day forum, David Stahl, chairman, held in New York City, December 1964. Contributors: Joseph M. Bail and others. Foreword by Harold P. Seligson. With descriptions and discussions of community crises in Savannah, Georgia, New York City, and Chester, Pennsylvania, 1963-1964.] N.Y., Practising Law Institute, 1966. 364 pp.

39. Pettigrew, Thomas Fraser. *A profile of the Negro American.* Princeton, N.J., London, Van Nostrand, 1964. 250 pp.

40. Silberman, Charles Eliot. *Crisis in black and white.* [Outgrowth of the author's articles "The City and the Negro" (*Fortune,* March 1962) and "The Businessman and the Negro" (*Fortune,* September 1963)] N.Y., Random House, 1964; London, Cape, 1965. 370 pp. Paperback ed.: N.Y., Vintage Books, 1964. 370 pp. (A Vintage book, V-279.)

41. *Families of the slums; an exploration of their structure and treatment,* by Salvador Minuchin, Braulio Montalvo, Bernard G. Guerney, Jr., Bernice L. Rosman, and Florence Schumer. [Outgrowth of a research project in family therapy conducted at the Wiltwyck School for Boys, a private residential treatment center for 100 boys, eight to twelve years of age. Based on work with twelve families, each of which had more than one delinquent child, and ten families which had no delinquent children. With case material and extensive excerpts from therapy sessions. With a review of the literature and bibliographies.] N.Y., Basic Books, 1967.

42. Lewis, Oscar. *La vida; a Puerto Rican family in the culture of poverty–San Juan and New York.* [The first of a series of volumes based upon a study of one hundred Puerto Rican families from four slums of Greater San Juan and of their relatives in New York City. Based on questionnaires, interviews, participant-observation, biographies, family case studies, and tests. With tape-recorded interviews, translated from Spanish into English.] N.Y., Random House, 1966. 669 pp. London, Secker & Warburg, 1967. 599 pp. Paperback ed.: N.Y., Vintage Books, a division of Random House, 1968. 669 pp. (A Vintage giant, V-421.)

43. Pavenstedt, Eleanor, ed. *The drifters: children of disorganized lower-class families,* by Charles A. Malone, Eleanor Pavenstedt, Ilse Mattick, Louise S. Bandler, Maurice R. Stein, and Norbett L. Mintz. [Based on the North Point Family Project, 1955-1959, undertaken under the auspices of the Boston University-Boston City Hospital Guidance Clinic in the Department of Child Psychiatry of the Division of Psychiatry, Boston University School of Medicine and on the North Point Demonstration Project, 1960-1965, representing intensive work with thirteen families and their forty-five pre-school children.] Foreword by Bernard Bandler. [With a survey of remedial programs for multiproblem families and their preschool children. With bibliographies.] Boston, Little, Brown; London, Churchill, 1967. 345 pp.

44. Wilensky, Harold L., and Lebeaux, Charles Nathan. *Industrial society and social welfare.* N.Y., Russell Sage Foundation, 1958. 401 pp. Paperback ed.: With a new introd. by Harold L. Wilensky.

N.Y., Free Press; London, Collier-Macmillan, 1965. 397 pp. (A Free Press paperback.)

45. Goldstein, Bernard. *Low income youth in urban areas; a critical review of the literature,* [primarily material published 1950-1966.] With the assistance of Barbara Steinberg and Harry C. Bredemeier. [Dedicated to Louis Wirth. With annotated references.] N.Y., London, Holt, Rinehart & Winston, 1967. 280 pp.

46. White, Mary Alice, and Charry, June, eds. *School disorder, intelligence, and social class.* [Report of a study of 2,866 pupil referrals to school psychologists, 1962-1963, designed and conducted by the Westchester Association of School Psychologists of New York State and a class in experimental school psychology, Teachers College, Columbia University. Based on questionnaires answered by 46 school psychologists representing 19 school systems in Westchester County. With a bibliography.] N.Y., Teachers College Press, 1966. 92 pp.

47. Lewis, Sir Aubrey Julian. *Inquiries in psychiatry: clinical and social investigations.* [Sixteen articles previously published, 1932-1963. Selected by the author's students to mark his retirement from the Maudsley Hospital in 1966. Companion volume to the author's *The state of psychiatry,* London, 1967. With case illustrations and bibliographies. With a complete bibliography of the author's publications, 1926-1966.] London, Routledge & Paul, 1967; N.Y., Science House, 1968, © 1967. 335 pp.

48. Lewis, Sir Aubrey Julian. *The state of psychiatry: essays and addresses* [previously published, 1934-1965. Edited by the author's students to mark his retirement from the Maudsley Hospital in 1966. Companion volume to the author's *Inquiries in psychiatry,* London, 1967. With reviews of the literature and bibliographies. With a complete bibliography of the author's publications, 1926-1966.] London, Routledge & Paul, 1967; N.Y., Science House, 1968, © 1967. 310 pp.

49. Allen, Gay Wilson. *William James; a biography.* [Based in part on unpublished letters and private diaries of William James and Alice Gibbens James. Dedicated to the memory of William James, 1882-1961. With a bibliography.] N.Y., Viking Press; London, Hart-Davis, 1967. 556 pp.

50. Friedman, Paul, ed. *On suicide, with particular reference to suicide among young students.* Discussions of the Vienna Psychoanalytic Society–1910. With contributions by Alfred Adler, Sigmund Freud [chairman], Josef K. Friedjung, Karl Molitor, David Ernst Oppenheim, Rudolf Reitler, J. [Isidor] Sadger, and Wilhelm Stekel. [Translated from the German, Wiener Psychoanalytische Vereinigung,

*Über den Selbstmord,* Wien, 1910, as a project of the Library Committee of the New York Psychoanalytic Institute. Translation first drafted by Edward Fitzgerald.] Edited [and with a historical review of the literature] by Paul Friedman. [Pref. by Alfred Adler. With case material.] N.Y., International Universities Press; London, Bailey & Swinfen [distributor], 1967. 121 pp.

# ESSAY 12

# *Lectureships in the Behavioral Sciences—An Introduction to Sociobibliography*

Originally published as Editorial in *Mental Health Book Review Index,* vol. 15 (whole no. 20), 1970.

## SEARCH FOR A LOST LITERATURE

For centuries the names of distinguished scientists and scholars have been linked with invited lectures endowed for a special purpose, yet little is known about the significance of this development. The lectureships, named after their founders or after persons to be honored, differ from university chairs in that the lecturers vary; and they differ from academic celebrations–such as the 20th anniversary of Clark University in 1909 where Freud gave his five lectures, "The Origin and Development of Psychoanalysis"–in that the lectures recur, usually every year, over long periods of time. In contrast to inaugural university lectures or adult-education lectures, invited lectures are often directed to both professional and lay audiences. In various ways the lectureships are intended to go beyond the ordinary, and in this lies their prestige. The lecturers share and sustain this prestige, often seizing the opportunity to probe deeply into a problem, to provide a synthesis, or to present a new idea. The selection committees exert a fundamental influence but usually remain in the background, even when they are identified. As they bestow the honor of an invitation, they must fulfill and reinterpret their trust and strike a balance between retrospective and current relevance, between continuity and change.

The literature that results from these lectures is likely to combine selectivity, concentration, and a sense of direction, to embody not so much the hard data of research as the humane thought of eminent scholars and scientists. Nevertheless, as the "literature of lectures" passes from its distinguished origins into the bibliographic record, it becomes itself less and less distinguishable.

In this editorial we discuss what might be gained by organizing these publications bibliographically by their form as lectures, in addition to their present bibliographic organization by subject matter. As an illustration, we present a brief bibliography of lectures published as books, or parts of books, that have been listed in the *Mental Health Book Review Index,* Volumes 1-15, 1956-1970. The list serves, therefore, to suggest the kinds of lectureships that are pertinent to the behavioral sciences, and it may help to raise the questions about the nature of these lectureships which a systematic study might then undertake to answer. This is a task for which social and bibliographic research must be joined. Such a new mode of inquiry, called "sociobibliography," would bring bibliographic data to bear on social studies and would modify the aims and methods of bibliography in the light of social research. This approach, though as yet without a basis in any discipline, has many potential applications to now neglected or seemingly insoluble problems. In the hope of contributing to such a development, we present this editorial as an introduction to sociobibliography.

## TYPES OF LECTURESHIPS–ORIGIN AND DEVELOPMENT

Lectureships are a meta-academic institution, dating from the dawn of modern science in the British Isles, and still continuing to flourish primarily in English-speaking countries. Perhaps more often through intuition than deliberate design, their most notable function, and the one of special interest today, may have been to resolve conflicts between an inert system and the changing needs of society. Important lectureships have achieved a liberalizing breakthrough by working from outside and yet with the "Establishment."

These eponymous lectureships, as they are sometimes called, developed first in the field of medicine. The four oldest, established at the

the most famous 19th-century lectureships in religion is easily apparent. In the Hibbert Lectures, first given in 1873 on terms inviting "the unfettered exercise of private judgment in matters of religion," specialists of international rank dealt with the history of the religions of the world. The Gifford Lectures, founded by a Scottish jurist who left £80,000 for a lectureship at each of the Scottish universities, Edinburgh, Glasgow, Aberdeen, and St. Andrews, allowed the freest research, without regard to tradition or established belief: the lecturers "may be of any religion or way of thinking or . . . they may be so-called skeptics or agnostics, or freethinkers," and they were to deal with Natural Theology as a "strictly natural science." Shortly after the turn of the century, the Silliman Memorial and the Terry Lectures at Yale University, while still reflecting a theological background, provided a forum for 20th-century scientific thought.

The founders of the lectureships first developed in the field of medicine have kept aloof from the university. They established lectureships within their own societies, where they were pursuing new scientific and professional goals. After journals came into existence, the majority of lectures given before professional and learned societies were published, if at all, as articles or only as abstracts. Most of the founders of the type of lectureships which has spread from theology to other fields, however, have been laymen with respect to the subject matter of the lectures. They have turned to the university and used its academic setting, although they themselves defined the terms of the endowment. Substantial amounts of money have been available to lecture foundations of this second type. Many of them support annual lecture series, and some enable a lecturer to reside at a university other than his own during an academic year or two and provide for publication of the lectures in the form of a book. Both types of lectures have been credited, however, with having been the medium for many of the classic expositions of their respective subjects, and both have led to contributions that broke new ground.

## LECTURES AS SOURCE MATERIAL ABOUT LECTURESHIPS

One of the characteristics of lectures is that they vary enormously, not only in the choice and treatment of topics, but also in many other ways. In their presentation, they are likely to be individual creations and, therefore, deserve to be studied as a form of scientific literature. Any published lecture may contain incidental information about lectures in general, and the lectureship under which it was delivered in particular. This information is, however, as elusive as many of the lectures themselves, and it is unpredictable whether or where salient data or comments will appear. They may be provided by the trustees, the lecturer, or the publisher. The first lecture in a series sometimes includes more and sometimes less of such information than later volumes. In the following, we will give a few illustrations of what lectures themselves contribute to a study of this form.

## THE MARK OF DISTINCTION

A great many lecturers begin by expressing their appreciation of the honor bestowed upon them and by explaining their own qualifications and approach. These remarks are often humble, but actually they reveal how broadly the trustees interpret the scope of the lectureship. A classic example is William James's introduction to his Gifford Lectures, *The Varieties of Religious Experience,* delivered at Edinburgh in 1901-1902. "It is with no small amount of trepidation that I take my place behind this desk, and face this learned audience," he began, and then he commented on the novelty "of talking whilst the Europeans listen," instead of listening whilst they talk, and suggested the exchange of lecturers in the future. He considered the appointment a "heroic obligation" which it would never do to decline, and described himself as neither a theologian, nor a scholar learned in the history of religions, nor an anthropologist. Psychology, he claimed, was the only branch of learning in which he was particularly versed. With his acknowledgment that his book would never have been written had he not been honored with this invitation, he made a point that applies to countless contributions to knowledge which lectureships have brought into existence. "When a man is chosen Harveian Orator," Sir Aubrey Lewis began his oration in 1963, "it sets him thinking about his fitness for this signal honour, considering the notable roll of those who have had it before him and the quality and value of what they said." Here, as well as in his 30th Hobhouse Memorial Lecture, he pointed out the recency and significance of having this honor bestowed upon a psychiatrist.

The terms of many lectureships are quite specific in requiring that the lecturers should be men or women "of distinction" on the stated subjects, "eminent scholars," "outstanding individuals." A particularly strong wording of this rather common clause appears in one of the James S. Carpentier Lectures. General Horace W. Carpentier, who established this lectureship at the Columbia University School of Law in 1903 in honor of his brother, expressed the desire that the lecturers be "chosen for pre-eminent fitness and ability" and that "this lectureship will be made so honorable that nobody, however great or distinguished, will willingly choose to decline your invitation."

## "AGENTS OF CULTURAL ADVANCE"

Concern with excellence is often coupled with efforts to integrate knowledge for the benefit of many. This view may be expressed by the lecturer himself. The late Lord Brain called the Riddell Memorial Lectures, which he delivered in 1958, "a memorial to a philosopher," noted his own "amateur status in philosophy," and continued: "but if the expanding universe of knowledge is not to carry all the specialists into ever-increasing isolation from each other, and the rest of the world, some attempt must be made here and there to achieve a comprehensive view. I have therefore tried to do this in the field of perception." Some lectureships are designed to achieve such integration. The Kappa Delta Pi Lecture Series was planned so that eventually it would "comprehend discussions by well known philosophers, scientists, educators and litterateurs whose combined interpretations of modern education should prove invaluable to professional and lay reader, alike." More emphatically, the deed of gift to Yale University for the Dwight Harrington Terry Foundation Lectures on Religion in the Light of Science and Philosophy sets forth the very broad range of the sciences and branches of knowledge that have a bearing on the subject, concluding that the lectures be given "to the end . . . that mankind may be helped to attain its highest possible welfare and happiness upon this earth."

The same deed declares that "the object of this foundation is not the promotion of scientific investigation and discovery, but rather the assimilation and interpretation of that which has been or shall be hereafter discovered." Two issues are raised here. One is that lectureships can themselves become "agents of cultural advance"—the title of Sir Aubrey Lewis's Hobhouse Memorial Lecture—by raising the level of understanding and cultural progress in the widest possible circles of the scientific community and society at large. The other is recognition of the need to keep the perspective open for the knowledge of the future. This insight is illustrated in the history of the Henderson Trust Lectures. The Trust was founded in 1832 for "the advancement and diffusion of the Science of Phrenology." The founder, however, foresaw that "what might seem of advantage then might not be advisable in the future." In the course of time, the trustees have arranged annual lectures on the development and function of the human brain, one of which is the one cited in our bibliography, O. L. Zangwill's *Cerebral Dominance and its Relation to Psychological Function.*

## ACADEMIC INNOVATIONS

Lectureships can not only transcend disciplines, but can also promote their convergence. For example, the Issac Ray Award, which was established in 1952 at the American Psychiatric Association in honor of the founder of forensic psychiatry in this country, is given annually to either a psychiatrist or a jurist who has already contributed "to the improvement of the relations of Law and Psychiatry." The recipient is expected to deliver the Isaac Ray Award Lectures at a university which has both a law school and a medical school. The books which resulted from these lectures, given at Harvard, Yale, Columbia, Michigan, Temple, Tulane, and a number of other universities, have dealt with topics that have since moved into the forefront of social issues.

Lectureships then bridge the earlier gap between scientific societies and universities. Another example is the eleven Walter Van Dyke Bingham Lectures on the Development of Exceptional Abilities and Capacities, recently collected by Dael Wolfle in a book, *The Discovery of Talent.* Delivered between 1954 and 1965 at different universities with the cooperation of the American Psychological Association, they were originally published in the Association's official organ, the *American Psychologist.* A trust can also cooperate with several universities, under whose auspices the lectures are given. The trustees of the Hamlyn Trust include representatives of the Universities of London, Wales, Leeds, Glasgow, Belfast, and Exeter. Lectureships may, therefore, set an example of interuniversity cooperation.

## SOCIAL ISSUES AND HUMAN VALUES

Lectures in the social sciences often try to relate scholarship to social progress: for example, the Florina Lasker Lectures of 1953 on "America's Role in International Social Welfare" are introduced with a call for "a science of international social welfare," and the John Dewey Society Lectureship opened in 1958 with Ordway Tead's lecture, "The Climate of Learning: a Constructive Attack on Complacency in Higher Education." In England, the Charles Russell Memorial Lecture honors the first Chief Inspector of Reformatory and Industrial Schools who, at the time of World War I, transformed their methods. The lectures on working-class and delinquent boys and girls are to reflect the spirit of his work.

Even the mere titles of lectures may throw light on the pace of social progress. In 1968, two officials of the Eugenics Society wrote concerning the Society's Galton Lectures: "In the light of recent events it is interesting to note that in 1942 Professor J. D. Bernal . . . spoke on 'The Need for a Social Sciences Research Council'; unfortunately, this was one of the few Galton Lectures which were not published." The comment referred by implication to the fact that such a Council was actually founded in England almost a quarter of a century later, in 1965. In the area of the social sciences, trustees and lecturers are often close to the social events of their time. These lectures can, therefore, become sources for social history as well as for the history of ideas. The Godkin Lectures on "The Essentials of Free Government and the Duties of the Citizen," established at Harvard in 1903, have from time to time reflected the challenges to these essentials. The Benjamin N. Cardozo Lectures of the Association of the Bar of the City of New York, which have, since their inception in 1941, included among their lecturers the Supreme Court Justices Jackson, Frankfurter, Douglas, Harlan, and Warren, have raised legal, constitutional, and social issues of widening public concern.

Lectures are often the most appropriate medium for examining the underlying philosophy of a field and, in particular, its relationships to values. This is illustrated in such titles as "The Law and Human Values" (Arthur T. Vanderbilt in the Pitcairn-Crabbe Lecture, 1951), "Psychiatry and Human Values" (John C. Whitehorn in the First Hamilton Memorial Lecture, 1953), and "Psychoanalysis and Moral Values" (Heinz Hartmann in the Freud Anniversary Lecture, 1959). A historical study would help to trace earlier phases of this trend and also lead to earlier relevant sources, for example, the John Calvin McNair Lectureship, inaugurated in 1908 at the University of North Carolina, which concerns the relationship between science and human values.

To be as significant in our time as they have been in previous centuries, lectureships should do more than cultivate new knowledge, even more than contribute to social enlightenment and reform: they should play a leading role with respect to the interlocking of science, society, and public affairs. That this is indeed happening is suggested, for example, by the George B. Pegram Lectureship. It provides for the lecturer's residence at Brookhaven National Laboratory and was established by the trustees of Associated Universities, Inc., as an opportunity "for reflective appraisal of the import of science on society by the very architects of current events and trends."

## CONTROVERSY AND CRITIQUE

The lecturers, though distinguished in their field, do not have "the last word." A well-known example of the controversy that may stem from a lecture is that which led from C. P. Snow's Rede Lecture of 1959, *The Two Cultures and the Scientific Revolution,* to the Richmond Lecture delivered in 1962 by his chief critic, F. R. Leavis, at the same university, Cambridge. The persons honored by an invitation to deliver a lecture appear to be very much aware of others who have given lectures in the recent or more distant past. Quotes and comments in one lecture referring to a previous one usually express consent or admiration and add a certain intimacy and continuity to the literature of lectures.

Adverse criticism has challenged lectures on the ground that their general purpose conflicts with the interests of specialization. For example, when Kenneth W. Spence published in 1956 his Silliman Memorial Lectures, *Behavior Theory and Conditioning,* he noted that he had been the first to represent psychology in this lecture series and described the specialist's dilemma "of presenting a series of lectures to an audience composed of laymen, scientists from other fields, and psychologists of all varieties of special interests and viewpoints." Louis Henry Jordan had earlier raised even stronger objections in his book *Comparative Religion,* a survey of the literature for the years 1900-1909. Although he had to acknowledge that this field owed a heavy debt to books produced under the auspices of lectureships, he felt nevertheless that lectureships "are not likely to furnish an adequate or permanent solution of the problem with which their generous founders are courageously grappling." He noted the risk that is "inseparable from the too rapid popularization" of such questions and stressed the need of "the founding of university *chairs,* competently manned." This criticism, however, misses a crucial point. To establish a new discipline is an exceedingly slow process. Lectureships help break the ground on which new academic curricula and departments can then be built.

When scientific and professional societies sponsor a lectureship, it is generally understood that the lectures will appear in the society's official organ. Only rarely does the lecturer himself submit his paper for editorial review; usually lectures published as articles are exempt from the reviewing process which guards the quality of the journal literature. Criticism can, however, follow their publication. For example, after William Sargant's Maudsley Lecture of 1968, "The Physiology of Faith," appeared in the May 1969 issue of the *British Journal of Psychiatry,* this journal published (November 1969) three letters to the Editor expressing doubts about the validity of the lecturer's arguments. The *Review of Religious Research* published first the H. Paul Douglass Lectures for 1969 by Milton Rokeach, and then a series of critiques by specialists from various fields together with the lecturer's reply (Fall 1969 and Winter 1970).

In theory, lectures which appear as books are subject to the usual evaluation through book reviews. In practice, however, certain inhibiting factors come into play here. University presses and nonprofit organizations which publish many lectures seldom use the techniques of book promotion as extensively as commercial publishers do. Furthermore, books derived from lectures may not easily fit into the scope of the specialized journals which are the media of book reviews for the scientific literature. This situation might change, if lectures were recognized and treated as a special form of scientific and scholarly writing.

## A PILOT BIBLIOGRAPHY OF LECTURES IN THE BEHAVIORAL SCIENCES

The bibliography that follows this essay includes all the lectures published as books or pamphlets which have been listed in the *Mental Health Book Review Index* since 1956. Almost half of the 124 lectures listed, and approximately one third of the 65 lectureships, were identified only through examining the books in which they appear, and more examples of this kind could probably be found. All the books listed were published between 1953 and 1968, but some contain lectures originally published much earlier in journals. Even the earliest lectureships, the Lumleian, Goulstonian, and Croonian Lectures and the Harveian Orations, are represented through lectures delivered during a period of almost a hundred years. There are also examples of lectureships inaugurated recently, between 1965 and 1967, within the behavioral sciences: the Langfeld Memorial and the Heinz Werner Lectures, established in psychology departments or institutes at universities, and the Hoch and the Hincks Memorial Lectures, founded by organizations in the fields of psychopathology and mental health.

The subjects span the whole range of the behavioral sciences, including the biomedical, psychological, and social sciences, the humanities, and the philosophy of science. Half of the lectureships were founded in the United States, half in the United Kingdom and Canada. More than half are under the auspices of learned societies, institutes, or trusts; the others are established at universities. The diversity in the media and formats of publication is amply illustrated. The bibliography constitutes, therefore, a small but representative sample of lectures pertinent to the behavioral sciences and delivered under currently active lectureships.

A list of the lecturers and lectureships precedes the bibliography.

## A STUDY IN SOCIOBIBLIOGRAPHY

As has been shown, the authors of lectures had previously gained recognition. Their topics are central to their own work or concerns, yet also of broader interest; and their presentations are usually directed to both learned and lay audiences. Lectures pertinent to the behavioral sciences should, therefore, be of particular value to those who seek a general orientation concerning the entire area for such purposes as teaching, the administration of research, and the design and evaluation of reference works, bibliographic services, and library collections. The need for such an orientation is hardly in doubt, especially since the name "behavioral sciences" is now freely applied to interdisciplinary activities of more limited scope. That lectures can serve as an aid for gaining a comprehensive view is, however, an assumption that needs to be validated through research. Taking the material presented here as a starting point, we suggest four pilot studies in sociobibliography and also mention a few by-products that may evolve.

1. *A core collection of lectures* in the behavioral sciences, which actually assembles the 124 lectures listed in our bibliography, would make it possible to examine them as forming a body of scientific literature. This collection would provide many leads for obtaining more complete information about these and similar lectureships. A comparative study of the characteristics of these publications would yield the data necessary for an informed proposal to develop a comprehensive bibliographic service responsible for tracing, listing, and indexing lectures in the behavioral sciences. A description of the diverse practices now in use would show the administrators and publishers of current lecture series, and the founders of new ones, what others have done. Such a survey would reveal what is exemplary in the design of lectureships and the dissemination of lectures, and would probably lead to improvements.

2. *A review of the book reviews* is, in this instance, a manageable task. The lectures listed appear in 100 books which have elicited some 600 reviews and critical book notes. The collective, multidisciplinary reviews of the published lectures no longer reflect only the expectations of the selection committees, but also the judgments of the reviewers who usually evaluate many other books in their respective fields. An analysis of these reviews should help greatly to determine the significance of the individual lectures. It may also lead to the formulation of standards for evaluating lectures by taking their special function in science and scholarship into account. Both the criticism and the criteria de-

rived from it should be useful to selection committees, lecturers, reviewers, and librarians.

3. *A historical study* of data further expanded from the first two studies should help to raise new questions, for example: at what point did lecturers and topics associated with the behavioral sciences become eligible for lectureships in the old established fields, mainly medicine, religion, and law? What is the history of lectureships founded in the 20th century under auspices already identified with the behavioral sciences, especially psychology, psychiatry, and psychoanalysis, and what has been their impact? Have these lectures significantly advanced the integration of knowledge in the behavioral sciences? What do lecture series, which consist of consecutive presentations by individual scientists and scholars, contribute to the communication of knowledge and the history of ideas as compared to other devices used by the scientific community, such as conferences and symposia? Are important lectures still landmarks, as were William James's Gifford Lectures, signaling new trends to follow in the wake of highly original work?

4. *A sociological study* would try to develop methods of social research for identifying lectureships in the biomedical, social, and psychological sciences. It would also gather new data about lectureships as a cultural phenomenon. This research should throw light on the manner in which lectureships are instituted and sustained. When a lectureship is established at a university, does the university then or later direct its course by extending the invitations, or does it mainly handle administrative matters? Plans for lectureships that cover some or all branches of knowledge usually follow the wishes of a wealthy donor; however, in the behavioral sciences—although not there alone—lectureships founded in honor of a person often provide continuity for his most significant contribution. Do these different conceptions and approaches, one coming from outside, the other from inside the scientific community, greatly affect the nature of the lectures? It appears that lectureships have been founded in large numbers at certain periods, for example, in the early 1900's and after World War II. Does this reflect a response to the influx of new knowledge, or the influence of socioeconomic factors, or the damaging effects of wars and depressions? What are the equivalents to endowed lectureships in the Western European countries which do not have them, and what else do these cultural differences signify?

Distinguished lecturers in the behavioral sciences will continue to be heard by many more than those they originally addressed, especially when they focus on areas of social and intellectual ferment. The literature formed by their lectures, however, needs further recognition, through studies which clarify the place of lectureships in science and society, and through bibliographies and library collections which keep their influence alive. It may be hoped that, with such bibliographic support, these lectures of our time can continue to reach their potential audiences and help them to attain broader views, deeper insights, and higher goals for the cultural advance of all men.

## A Bibliography of 124 Lectures in 65 Lectureships Derived from the Selective Listings of Books in the *Mental Health Book Review Index*, Volumes 1-15, 1956-1970

Part 1. List of Lecturers and Lectureships

| *Lecturer* | *Lectureship* |
|---|---|
| Alexander, Franz | Hamilton |
| Allport, Gordon Willard | Morrison |
| Allport, Gordon Willard | Terry |
| Altmeyer, Arthur J. | Lasker |
| Arendt, Hannah | Walgreen |
| Bailey, Percival | Harris |
| Banton, Michael Parker | Munro |
| Baruk, Henri | Rees |
| Bertalanffy, Ludwig von | Werner |
| Biggs, John, Jr. | Ray |
| Bowman, Karl Murdock | Hamilton |
| Brain, Sir Walter Russell | Riddell |
| Burt, Cyril Lodowic | Clark |
| Carstairs, George Morris | Reith |
| Chisholm, Brock | Bampton |
| Clark, Sir Wilfrid Edward Le Gros | Munro |
| Cobb, Stanley | Hamilton |
| Denny-Brown, Derek Ernest | Croonian |
| Dobzhansky, Theodosius Grigorievich | Silliman |
| Dubos, René Jules | Pegram |
| Farnsworth, Dana Lyda | Salmon |
| Felix, Robert Hanna | Bampton |
| Freud, Anna | Freud |

| *Lecturer* | *Lectureship* |
|---|---|
| Gerard, Ralph Waldo | Morrison |
| Gibb, Jack R. | Morrison |
| Glueck, Bernard, Sr. | Hamilton |
| Glueck, Sheldon | Ray |
| Goffman, Erving | MacIver |
| Gombrich, Ernst Hans Josef | Mellon |
| Granit, Ragnar | Silliman |
| Greenacre, Phyllis | Freud |
| Guilford, Joy Paul | Bingham |
| Hargreaves, George Ronald | Clark |
| Hartmann, Heinz | Freud |
| Hartung, Frank E. | Martin |
| Hayakawa, Samuel Ichiyé | Morrison |
| Hilgard, Ernest Ropiequet | Morrison |
| Hoch, Paul Henry | Hamilton |
| Hoffer, Willi | Flexner |
| Holmes, Sir Gordon Morgan | Croonian |
| Horder, Sir Thomas Jeeves Horder | Harben |
| Huxley, Aldous Leonard | Morrison |
| Jackson, John Hughlings | Bowman |
| Jackson, John Hughlings | Croonian |
| Jackson, John Hughlings | Goulstonian |
| Jackson, John Hughlings | Hunterian |
| Jackson, John Hughlings | Jackson |
| Jackson, John Hughlings | Lumleian |
| Jervis, George Amedee | Hamilton |
| Jones, Ernest | Freud |
| Kallmann, Franz Josef | Hamilton |
| Kallmann, Franz Josef | Salmon |
| Kelman, Herbert C. | Morrison |
| Klüver, Heinrich | Hamilton |
| Koch, Sigmund | Morrison |
| Kubie, Lawrence Schlesinger | Porter |
| Lee, Roy Stuart | Burroughs |
| Leighton, Alexander Hamilton | Salmon |
| Levy, David Mordecai | Hamilton |
| Lewin, Bertram David | Freud |
| Lewis, Sir Aubrey Julian | Bradshaw |
| Lewis, Sir Aubrey Julian | Galton |
| Lewis, Sir Aubrey Julian | Harveian |
| Lewis, Sir Aubrey Julian | Hobhouse |

| *Lecturer* | *Lectureship* |
|---|---|
| Lewis, Sir Aubrey Julian | Manson |
| Lewis, Sir Aubrey Julian | Maudsley |
| Lewis, Sir Aubrey Julian | Meyer |
| Lewis, Sir Aubrey Julian | Roberts |
| Lewis, Nolan Don Carpentier | Hamilton |
| Lidz, Theodore | Sheckman |
| Linton, Ralph | Salmon |
| Magoun, Horace Winchell | Salmon |
| Maslow, Abraham Harold | Dewey Society |
| Maslow, Abraham Harold | Kappa Delta Pi |
| Maslow, Abraham Harold | Morrison |
| Mather, Kenneth | Matthews |
| Mead, Margaret | Terry |
| Medawar, Peter Brian | Reith |
| Menninger, Karl Augustus | Ray |
| Meyer, Adolf | Salmon |
| Murphy, Gardner | Dewey Society |
| Murphy, Gardner | Morrison |
| Myrdal, Alva Reiner, and others | Lasker |
| Newcomb, Theodore Mead | Morrison |
| Nunberg, Herman | Brill |
| Osgood, Charles Egerton | Morrison |
| Overholser, Winfred | Ray |
| Penfield, Wilder | Vanuxem |
| Piaget, Jean | Werner |
| Rado, Sandor | Hamilton |
| Radzinowicz, Leon | Carpentier |
| Rasey, Marie I., ed. | Franklin |
| Richter, Curt Paul | Hamilton |
| Riesman, David | Dewey Memorial |
| Roberts, Charles A. | Hincks |
| Roche, Philip Quintin | Ray |
| Rogers, Carl Ransom | Morrison |
| Rusk, Dean | Lasker |
| Sargant, William Walters | Smith |
| Shryock, Richard Harrison | Phelps |
| Smith, Henry Lee, Jr. | Inglish |
| Snow, Sir Charles Percy | Rede |
| Spence, Kenneth Wartenbee | Silliman |
| Spitz, René Arpad | Freud |
| Sprott, Walter John Herbert | Mason |

Royal College of Physicians of London, have continued to the present. For the Lumleian Lectures, which began in 1582, the appointment was originally for life, and in this they resembled a university chair outside the university. William Harvey, who was Lumleian Lecturer from 1616 to 1656, is supposed in this capacity to have expounded his new view of the circulation of the blood. In the Goulstonian Lectures, which began on an annual basis in 1639 with a bequest of £200, the lecturer was to be one of the four youngest doctors of the College. Harvey himself founded the Harveian Orations in 1656. Originally delivered in Latin, they were to exhort the fellows and members of the College "to search and study out the secrets of nature by way of experiment; and also for the honour of the profession to continue in mutual love and affection among themselves." A recent historian of the Royal College of Physicians, Sir George Clark, suggests that from the Harveian Orations—apparently the first lectures to be printed, though irregularly, beginning in 1661—"the learned world could judge how the College maintained its standards of civilized intellectual intercourse and professional service." Dr. Croone designed a plan, but left no money, for two lectureships, one for the Royal College of Physicians, the other for the Royal Society. When the plans were implemented later, both series were called Croonian Lectures.

The early lectureships in medicine reflected the need for a wider education for physicians and surgeons in the light of an increased knowledge of anatomy, Harveian physiology, and advances in physics and chemistry in the 17th century. The initiative came from fellows of the Royal College of Physicians. With their designs and endowments of lectureships, they encouraged a form of "continuing education" and enhanced the prestige of their institution, a pattern that has since been followed by innumerable professional organizations.

A different type of lectureship developed in the field of religion. The scientist Robert Boyle, one of the founders of the Royal Society in 1662, left an endowment for the first theological lectureship in 1691. These Boyle Lectures "for proving the Christian Religion against Notorious Infidels, namely, Atheists, Pagans, Jews, and Mahometans," and the Bampton Lectures instituted in similar terms at the University of Oxford in 1780, also set a lasting pattern. Often under denominational control, many such lectureships were established to support a particular type of theology. Against this background, the significance of

| *Lecturer* | *Lectureship* |
|---|---|
| Stone, Leo | Freud |
| Stürup, Georg Kristoffer | Ciba |
| Stürup, Georg Kristoffer | Ray |
| Sullivan, Harry Stack | White |
| Taylor, Harold | Morrison |
| Terman, Lewis Madison | Bingham |
| Trilling, Lionel | Freud |
| Von Békésy, Georg | Langfeld |
| Waelder, Robert | Freud |
| Walker, Nigel | Russell |
| Wall, William Douglas | National Children's Home |
| Washburn, Sherwood Larned | Ciba |
| Weihofen, Henry | Ray |
| White, Victor | Cadbury |
| Whitehorn, John Clare | Hamilton |
| Williams, Glenville Llewelyn | Carpentier |
| Wootton, Barbara | Hamlyn |
| Wootton, Barbara | Hoch |
| Young, John Zachary | Withering |
| Zangwill, Oliver Louis | Henderson |
| Zilboorg, Gregory | Ray |

## EXPLANATION OF THE FORMAT OF THE BIBLIOGRAPHY

The bibliography lists the lectureships, arranged alphabetically by the identifying surnames, together with the institutions at which they are established. The entries for the lectures give author, title, and year of publication. The serial number within a lecture series and/or the year when the lecture was given appear at the left. Several lectures in the same series are arranged chronologically.

Part 2. Bibliography

Bampton Lectures in America. Columbia University.

No. 10. 1957. Chisholm, Brock. *Prescription for survival.* N.Y., Columbia Univ. Pr., 1957; London, Oxford Univ. Pr., 1958. 92 pp. (Bampton lectures in America, no. 10.)

No. 16. 1965. Felix, Robert Hanna. *Mental illness; progress and prospects.* [With a bibliography.] N.Y., London, Columbia Univ. Pr., 1967. 110 pp. (Bampton lectures in America, no. 16.)

The Walter Van Dyke Bingham Lectures on the Development of Exceptional Abilities and Capacities. American Psychological Association.

1st. 1954. Terman, Lewis Madison. The discovery and encouragement of exceptional talent. *In* Jackson, Douglas Northrop, and Messick, Samuel, eds. *Problems in human assessment.* [Papers previously published, 1944-1964, with commentary. Dedicated to the memory of Irving Lorge, Edward K. Strong, Lewis M. Terman, and Louis Leon Thurstone. With reviews of the literature and bibliographies.] N.Y., London, McGraw-Hill, 1967. 873 pp. (McGraw-Hill series in psychology.) pp. 469-479.

6th. 1959. Guilford, Joy Paul. Three faces of intellect. *Ibid.,* pp. 421-433. *Also in* Nunnally, Jum Clarence. *Psychometric theory.* [With two previously published articles by Thelma G. Thurstone, 1941, and J. P. Guilford, 1959. With bibliographies.] N.Y., London, McGraw-Hill, 1967. 640 pp. (McGraw-Hill series in psychology.) pp. 448-468.

Bowman Lectures. Ophthalmological Society, London.

1885. Jackson, John Hughlings. Opthalmology and diseases of the nervous system. *In* Jackson, John Hughlings. *Selected writings.* Ed. for the guarantors of "Brain" by James Taylor, with the advice and assistance of Gordon Holmes and F. M. R. Walshe. 1st ed., 1931, reprinted. N.Y., Basic Books, 1958; London, Staples Press, 1959. 2 v. Vol. 2. pp. 346-358.

Bradshaw Lectures. Royal College of Physicians of London.

1957. Lewis, Sir Aubrey Julian. Between guesswork and certainty in psychiatry. *In* Lewis, Sir Aubrey Julian. *The state of psychiatry: essays and addresses* [previously published, 1934-1965. Edited by the author's students to mark his retirement from the Maudsley Hospital in 1966. Companion volume to the author's *Inquiries in psychiatry,* London, 1967. With reviews of the literature and bibliographies. With a complete bibliography of the author's publications, 1926-1966.] London, Routledge & Paul, 1967; N.Y., Science House, 1968, ©1967. 310 pp. Pp. 195-213.

Brill Memorial Lectures. New York Psychoanalytic Society.

11th. 1959. Nunberg, Herman. The Minutes of the Vienna Psychoanalytic Society—an introduction. *In* Wiener Psychoanalytische Vereinigung. *Minutes of the Vienna Psychoanalytic Society.* Vol. 1: 1906-1908. Ed. by Herman Nunberg and Ernst Federn. Transl. by M. Nunberg. N.Y., International Universities Press, 1962. 410 pp. Pp. xvii-xxxii.

Burroughs Memorial Lectures. Anglican Evangelical Group Movement, Central Committee and University of Leeds.

1953. Lee, Roy Stuart. *Psychology and worship.* London, SCM Press, 1955; N.Y., Philosophical Library, 1956. 110 pp. (Burroughs memorial lectures, 1953.)

Edward Cadbury Lectureship in Theology. University of Birmingham.

1958-1959. White, Victor. *Soul and psyche; an enquiry into the relationship of psychotherapy and religion.* N.Y., Harper; London, Collins & Harvill Press, 1960. 312 pp. (Edward Cadbury lectures, 1958-1959.)

James S. Carpentier Lectures. Columbia University School of Law.

15th ser. 1956. Williams, Glanville Llewelyn. *The sanctity of life and the criminal law;* an expanded and revised version of a series of five lectures delivered at the Columbia University School of Law in April 1956. With a foreword by William C. Warren. N.Y., Knopf, 1957. 350 pp. (Columbia University. School of Law. James S. Carpentier lectures, 15th ser., 1956) London, Faber & Faber, 1957. 319 pp.

1965. Radzinowicz, Leon. *Ideology and crime.* [James S. Carpentier lectures delivered at the Columbia University School of Law, 1965. Foreword by William C. Warren. With a bibliography.] N.Y., Columbia Univ. Pr., 1966. 152 pp. (James S. Carpentier lectures, 1965) British ed. with subtitle: *A study of crime in its social and historical context.* London, Heinemann, 1966. 152 pp. (James S. Carpentier lectures, 1965.)

Ciba Foundation Annual Lecture.

17th. 1965. Washburn, Sherwood Larned. Conflict in primate society. *In* De Reuck, Anthony V. S., and Knight, Julie, eds. *Conflict in society;* a Ciba Foundation volume. [Proceedings of a symposium arranged by the Ciba Foundation and held June 28-July 1, 1965 in London. Chairman's introd. by Alex Haddow. Members of the symposium: Zevedei Barbu and others. With the Ciba Foundation annual lecture, 1965: Conflict in primate society, by S. L. Washburn. Published in association with the International Peace Research Association. With bibliographies.] Boston, Little, Brown; London, Churchill, 1966. 467 pp. Pp. 3-15.

19th. 1967. Stürup, Georg Kristoffer. Will this man be dangerous? *In Symposium on the Mentally Abnormal Offender, London, 1967.* The mentally abnormal offender; a Ciba Foundation symposium, [Sir Charles Cunningham, chairman. Program devised by Henry Rollin and Nigel Walker.] Edited by A. V. S. de Reuck and Ruth Porter. [Membership of the symposium: E. Bittner and others. With the Ciba Foundation 19th annual lecture, 1967: Will this man be dangerous? by Georg K. Stürup. With reviews of the literature and bibliographies.] Boston, Little, Brown; London, Churchill, 1968. 260 pp. Pp. 5-18.

Heath Clark Lectures. London School of Hygiene and Tropical Medicine, University of London.

1933. Burt, Cyril Lodowic. *The subnormal mind.* 3d ed. N.Y., London, Oxford Univ. Pr., 1955. 391 pp. (University of London, Heath Clark lectures, 1933, delivered at the London School of Hygiene and Tropical Medicine.)

1957. Hargreaves, George Ronald. *Psychiatry and the public health.* N.Y., London, Oxford Univ. Pr., 1958. 118 pp. (London. University. London School of Hygiene and Tropical Medicine. Heath Clark lectures, 1957.)

Croonian Lectures. Royal College of Physicians of London.

1884. Jackson, John Hughlings. Evolution and dissolution of the nervous system. *In* Jackson, John Hughlings. *Selected writings.* Ed. for the guarantors of "Brain" by James Taylor, with the advice and assistance of Gordon Holmes and F. M. R. Walshe. 1st ed., 1931, reprinted. N.Y., Basic Books, 1958; London, Staples Press, 1959. 2 v. Vol. 2. Pp. 45-75.

1922. Holmes, Sir Gordon Morgan. The Croonian lectures on the clinical symptoms of cerebellar disease and their interpretation. *In* Holmes, Sir Gordon Morgan. *Selected papers of Sir Gordon Holmes.* Comp. and ed. by F. M. R. Walshe. Dedicated to Sir Gordon Holmes in homage on the occasion of his eightieth birthday by the guarantors of "Brain." N.Y., St. Martin's Press; London, Macmillan, 1956. Pp. 49-111.

1960. Denny-Brown, Derek Ernest. *The basal ganglia and their relation to disorders of movement.* [Croonian lectures, Royal College of Physicians of London, February 1960.] N.Y., London, Oxford Univ. Pr., 1962. 144 pp. (Oxford neurological monographs.)

John Dewey Memorial Lecture. Bennington College.

3rd. 1956. Riesman, David. Some continuities and discontinuities in the education of women. *In* Riesman, David. *Abundance for what?* And other essays [published or given as lectures 1954-1963. Dedicated to Erich Fromm.] Garden City, N.Y., Doubleday; London, Chatto & Windus, 1964. 610 pp. Pp. 307-330. Paperback ed.: Garden City, N.Y., Anchor Books, Doubleday, 1965. 579 pp. (A Doubleday anchor book, A473.)

The John Dewey Society Lectureship Series. John Dewey Society and National Society of College Teachers of Education.

No. 4. 1961. Murphy, Gardner. *Freeing intelligence through teaching;*

*a dialectic of the rational and the personal.* Foreword by Arthur G. Wirth. N.Y., London, Harper, 1961. 64 pp. (The John Dewey Society lectureship series, no. 4.)

No. 8. 1965. Maslow, Abraham Harold. *The psychology of science; a reconnaissance.* [A continuation of the author's *Motivation and personality,* N.Y., 1954. Series editor's] foreword by Arthur G. Wirth. [With a bibliography.] N.Y., London, Harper & Row, 1966. 168 pp. (The John Dewey Society lectureship series, no. 8.)

The Abraham Flexner Lectures Series. Vanderbilt University School of Medicine.

Ser. no. 12. 1953. Hoffer, Willi. *Psychoanalysis, practical and research aspects.* Baltimore, Williams & Wilkins; London, Baillière, 1955. 102 pp. (Vanderbilt University. School of Medicine. Abraham Flexner lectures. Series no. 12.)

The Leo M. Franklin Lectures in Human Relations. Wayne State University.

1956-1957. Vol. 6. Rasey, Marie I., ed. *The nature of being human.* Pref. by J. Wilmer Menge. Detroit, Wayne State Univ. Pr., 1959. 115 pp. (Leo M. Franklin lectures in human relations, 1956-1957.)

The Freud Anniversary Lecture Series. New York Psychoanalytic Institute.

4th. 1954. Freud, Anna. Psychoanalysis and education. *In The Psychoanalytic study of the child.* Vol. 9. Ed. by Anna Freud and others. N.Y., International Universities Press, 1954; London, Imago, 1955. 380 pp. Pp. 9-15. [Author's abstract.]

5th. 1955. Trilling, Lionel. *Freud and the crisis of our culture.* Based on the fifth Freud anniversary lecture, the New York Psychoanalytic Institute, 1955. Boston, Beacon Press, 1955. 59 pp. (Mid-century essays. no. 1.)

6th. 1956. Jones, Ernest. The nature of genius. *In* Jones, Ernest. *Sigmund Freud;* four centenary addresses. N.Y., Basic Books, 1956. 150 pp. Pp. 1-34.

7th. 1957. Lewin, Bertram David. *Dreams and the uses of regression.* N.Y., International Universities Press, 1958. 64 pp. (Freud anniversary lecture series, the New York Psychoanalytic Institute, 1957.)

8th. 1958. Spitz, René Arpad. *A genetic field theory of ego formation; its implications for pathology.* [An expanded version of the lecture held at the New York Academy of Medicine on May 27, 1958, under the title "Field theory of ego formation and its implications for pathology."] N.Y., International Universities Press; London, Bailey & Swinfen, 1959. 123 pp. (The Freud anniversary lecture series, 1958.)

9th. 1959. Hartmann, Heinz. *Psychoanalysis and moral values.* [An expanded version of the lecture given at the New York Academy of Medicine on May 12, 1959.] N.Y., International Universities Press; London, Bailey & Swinfen, 1960. 121 pp. (The Freud anniversary lecture series, the New York Psychoanalytic Institute, 1959.)

11th. 1961. Stone, Leo. *The psychoanalytic situation: an examination of its development and essential nature.* [An expanded version of the lecture given at the New York Academy of Medicine on May 9, 1961.] N.Y., International Universities Press, 1962, © 1961. 160 pp. (The Freud anniversary lecture series, the New York Psychoanalytic Institute. 1961.)

12th. 1962. Greenacre, Phyllis. *The quest for the father; a study of the Darwin-Butler controversy, as a contribution to the understanding of the creative individual.* [An expanded version of the lecture given at the New York Academy of Medicine, May 22, 1962.] N.Y., International Universities Press; London, Bailey & Swinfen [distributor], 1963. 128 pp. (The Freud anniversary lecture series of the New York Psychoanalytic Institute, 1962.)

13th. 1963. Waelder, Robert. *Psychoanalytic avenues to art.* [An expanded version of the lecture given at the New York Academy of Medicine on May 21, 1963. With a bibliography and a list of the author's publications, 1924-1965.] N.Y., International Universities Press, 1965. 122 pp. (The Freud anniversary lecture series of the New York Psychoanalytic Institute, 1963.) London, Hogarth Press and Institute of Psycho-Analysis, 1965. 122 pp. (The Freud anniversary lecture series of the New York Psychoanalytic Institute, 1963. Psychoanalytical epitomes, no. 6.)

Galton Lectures. Eugenics Society, London.

1958. Lewis, Sir Aubrey Julian. Fertility and mental illness. *In* Lewis, Sir Aubrey Julian. *Inquiries in psychiatry: clinical and social investigations.* [Sixteen articles previously published, 1932-1963. Selected by the author's students to mark his retirement from the Maudsley Hospital in 1966. Companion volume to the author's *The state of psychiatry,* London, 1967. With case illustrations and bibliographies. With a complete bibliography of the author's publications, 1926-1966.] London, Routledge & Paul, 1967; N.Y., Science House, 1968, ©1967. 335 pp. Pp. 285-305.

Goulstonian Lectures. Royal College of Physicians of London.

1869. Jackson, John Hughlings. Certain points in the study and classification of diseases of the nervous system. [Abstract.] *In* Jackson, John Hughlings. *Selected writings.* Ed. for the guarantors of "Brain" by James Taylor, with the advice and assistance of Gordon Holmes and F. M. R. Walshe. 1st ed., 1931, reprinted. N.Y., Basic Books, 1958; London, Staples Press, 1959. 2 v. Vol. 2. Pp. 246-250.

The Samuel W. Hamilton Memorial Lecture. American Psychopathological Association.

1953. Whitehorn, John Clare. Psychiatry and human values. *In* Hoch, Paul Henry, and Zubin, Joseph, eds. *Psychiatry and the law.* N.Y., Grune & Stratton, 1955. 232 pp. (American Psychopathological Association. Proceedings of the annual meeting. 43d, 1953.) Pp. 144-156.

1954. Levy, David Mordecai. Oppositional syndromes and oppositional behavior. *In* Hoch, Paul Henry, and Zubin,

Joseph, eds. *Psychopathology of childhood.* N.Y., Grune & Stratton, 1955; London, Heinemann, 1956. 303 pp. (American Psychopathological Association. Proceedings of the annual meeting. 44th, 1954.) Pp. 204-226.

1955. Cobb, Stanley. Awareness, attention and physiology of the brain stem. *In* Hoch, Paul Henry, and Zubin, Joseph, eds. *Experimental psychopathology.* N.Y., Grune & Stratton; London, Heinemann, 1957. 275 pp. (American Psychopathological Association. Proceedings of the annual meeting. 45th, 1955.) Pp. 194-204.

1956. Rado, Sandor. Psychotherapy: a problem of controlled inter-communication. *In* Hoch, Paul Henry, and Zubin, Joseph, eds. *Psychopathology of communication.* N.Y., Grune & Stratton; London, Heinemann, 1958. 305 pp. (American Psychopathological Association. Proceedings of the annual meeting. 46th, 1956.) Pp. 214-226.

1957. Bowman, Karl Murdock. Some problems of addiction. *In* Hoch, Paul Henry, and Zubin, Joseph, eds. *Problems of addiction and habituation.* N.Y., London, Grune & Stratton, 1958. 250 pp. (American Psychopathological Association. Proceedings of the annual meeting. 47th, 1957.) Pp. 161-176.

1958. Glueck, Bernard, Sr. Psychoanalysis: reflections and comments. *In* Hoch, Paul Henry, and Zubin, Joseph, eds. *Current approaches to psychoanalysis.* N.Y., London, Grune & Stratton, 1960. 207 pp. (American Psychopathological Association. Proceedings of the annual meeting. 48th, 1958.) Pp. 123-140.

1960. Kallmann, Franz Josef. Genetic factors in aging: comparative and longitudinal observations on a senescent twin population. *In* Hoch, Paul Henry, and Zubin, Joseph, eds. *Psychopathology of aging.* N.Y., London, Grune & Stratton, 1961. 321 pp. (American Psychopathological Association. Proceedings of the annual meeting. 50th, 1960.) Pp. 227-247.

1961. Lewis, Nolan Don Carpentier. Reflections on the past, present and future of psychiatric progress. *In* Hoch, Paul Henry, and Zubin, Joseph, eds. *The future of psychiatry.* N.Y., London, Grune & Stratton, 1962. 271 pp. (American Psychopathological Association. Proceedings of the annual meeting. 51st, 1961.) Pp. 147-181.

1962. Alexander, Franz. Evaluation of psychotherapy. *In* Hoch, Paul Henry, and Zubin, Joseph, eds. *The evaluation of psychiatric treatment;* the proceedings of the Fifty-second Annual Meeting of the American Psychopathological Association held in New York City, February 1962. [With an introd.: Franz Alexander, M.D., Samuel W. Hamilton, award lecturer, 1962, by Paul H. Hoch. With the Samuel W. Hamilton award lecture for 1962: Evaluation of psychotherapy, by Franz Alexander. Lillian and Henry Stratton award for the 1962 Symposium: Heinz E. Lehmann. With bibliographies.] N.Y., London, Grune & Stratton, 1964. 326 pp. Pp. 176-193.

1963. Klüver, Heinrich. Neurobiology of normal and abnormal perception. *In* Hoch, Paul Henry, and Zubin, Joseph, eds. *Psychopathology of perception;* the proceedings of the Fifty-third Annual Meeting of the American Psychopathological Association, held in New York City, February 1963. [With an introd.: Heinrich Klüver, Samuel W. Hamilton memorial lecturer, by Paul C. Bucy. With the Samuel W. Hamilton award lecture for 1963: Neurobiology of normal and abnormal perception, by Heinrich Klüver. Lillian and Henry Stratton award for the 1963 Symposium: Charles W. Eriksen and Ronald Melzack.] N.Y., London, Grune & Stratton, 1965. 336 pp. Pp. 1-40.

1964. Hoch, Paul Henry. Schizophrenia. *In* Hoch, Paul Henry, and Zubin, Joseph, eds. *Psychopathology of schizophrenia;* the proceedings of the Fifty-fourth Annual Meeting of the American Psychopathological Association held in New York City, February 1964. [With an introd.: Paul H. Hoch, M.D., Hamilton memorial award lecturer, 1964, by Jerome D. Frank. With the Samuel W. Hamilton memorial award lecture for 1964:

Schizophrenia, by Paul H. Hoch. Henry M. and Lillian Stratton awards for the 1964 Symposium: Robert W. Payne and Kurt Salzinger. With the presidential address by Jerome D. Frank: Contributions of behavioral scientists toward a world without war, previously published in *Comprehensive Psychiatry,* 1964. With case reports, a historical review of the literature, and bibliographies.] N.Y., London, Grune & Stratton, 1966. 582 pp. Pp. 283-301.

1965. Richter, Curt Paul. Psychopathology of periodic behavior in animals and man. *In* Zubin, Joseph, and Hunt, Howard Francis, eds. *Comparative psychopathology: animal and human;* the proceedings of the Fifty-fifth Annual Meeting of the American Psychopathological Association, held in New York City, February 1965. [With an introductory sketch: Curt P. Richter, Samuel W. Hamilton memorial lecturer, 1965, by Lawrence C. Kolb. With the Samuel W. Hamilton memorial award lecture for 1965: Psychopathology of periodic behavior in animals and man, by Curt P. Richter. Henry M. and Lillian Stratton award: David A. Rodgers. With reports and reviews of research and bibliographies.] N.Y., Grune & Stratton; London, Heinemann Medical Books [distributor], 1967. 350 pp. Pp. 205-227.

1966. Jervis, George Amedee. Some observations on the problem of heredity and environment in mental retardation. *In* Zubin, Joseph, and Jervis, George Amedee, eds. *Psychopathology of mental development;* the proceedings of the Fifty-sixth Annual Meeting of the American Psychopathological Association, held in New York City, February 1966. [With an introductory sketch: George A. Jervis, Samuel W. Hamilton memorial lecturer, 1966, by Elaine F. Kinder. With the Samuel W. Hamilton memorial award lecture for 1966: Some observations on the problem of heredity and environment in mental retardation, by George A. Jervis. With the presidential address by Seymour S. Kety: Intelligence, biology and social responsibility. With reviews of the literature and bibliographies.] N.Y., Grune & Stratton; London, Heinemann Medical Books [distributor], 1967. 658 pp. Pp. 262-269.

Hamlyn Lectures. Hamlyn Trust.

15th ser. 1963. Wootton, Barbara Adam. *Crime and the criminal law; reflections of a magistrate and social scientist.* [With a foreword: The Hamlyn Trust by John Murray.] Published under the auspices of the Hamlyn Trust. London, Stevens, 1963. 118 pp. (The Hamlyn lectures, 15th ser.)

The Harben Lectures. Royal Institute of Public Health, London.

1952. Horder, Thomas Jeeves Horder. *Fifty years of medicine.* An expanded version of the Harben lectures, 1952. London, Duckworth, 1953; N.Y., Philosophical Library, 1954. 70 pp.

The Norman Wait Harris Lectures. Norman Wait Harris Foundation. Northwestern University.

1963. Bailey, Percival. *Sigmund the unserene: a tragedy in three acts.* [Three essays on Sigmund Freud.] With a foreword by Roy R. Grinker, Sr. [The Norman Wait Harris lectures given at Northwestern University on April 15, 16, 18, 1963. With a bibliography.] Springfield, Ill., Thomas, 1965. 127 pp.

The Harveian Oration. Royal College of Physicians of London.

1963. Lewis, Sir Aubrey Julian. Medicine and the affections of the mind. *In* Lewis, Sir Aubrey Julian. *The state of psychiatry: essays and addresses* [previously published, 1934-1965. Edited by the author's students to mark his retirement from the Maudsley Hospital in 1966. Companion volume to the author's *Inquiries in psychiatry,* London, 1967. With reviews of the literature and bibliographies. With a complete bibliography of the author's publications, 1926-1966.] London, Routledge & Paul, 1967; N.Y., Science House, 1968, © 1967; 310 pp. Pp. 273-294.

The Henderson Trust Lectures. William Ramsay Henderson Trust, Edinburgh.

No. 19. Zangwill, Oliver Louis. *Cerebral dominance and its relation to psychological function.* Edinburgh, Publ. for the William Ramsay Henderson Trust by Oliver & Boyd, 1960. 31 pp. (Henderson Trust lectures, no. 19.)

Clarence M. Hincks Memorial Lectures. Ontario Mental Health Foundation, Toronto.

1st. 1967. Roberts, Charles A. Primary prevention of psychiatric disorders. *In Primary prevention of psychiatric disorders:* the [first] Clarence M. Hincks memorial lectures, [delivered at the University of Ottawa, February 2, 3, and 4,] 1967, by C. A. Roberts; including Medical aspects of primary prevention of psychiatric disorders, papers presented at the University of Ottawa, [at the postgraduate conference of the Faculty of Medicine on "Primary Prevention of Psychiatric Disorders," held on] February (2-4,) 1967, by W. Harding Le Riche, Morton Beiser, R. C. A. Hunter, John A. Rassell, Benjamin Goldberg, V. A. Kral, A. Lamberti, D. G. McKerracher, J. D. Griffin, and V. Szyrinski. Edited by F. C. R. Chalke and J. J. Day. [Foreword by Arthur Kelly. With a biographical sketch: Clarence Meredith Hincks, B.A., M.D., D.Sc., LL.D., 1885-1964. With an introductory statement: Dr. Charles A. Roberts, Hincks memorial lecturer, 1967. With bibliographies.] Toronto, Published for the Ontario Mental Health Foundation by Univ. of Toronto Pr.; London, Oxford Univ. Pr. [distributor], 1968. 168 pp. (Clarence M. Hincks memorial lectures, 1967.) Pp. 1-66.

L. T. Hobhouse Memorial Trust Lecture. London University.

30th. 1960. Lewis, Sir Aubrey Julian. Agents of cultural advance. *In* Lewis, Sir Aubrey Julian. *The state of psychiatry: essays and addresses* [previously published, 1934-1965. Edited by the author's students to mark his retirement from the Maudsley Hospital in 1966. Companion volume to the author's *Inquiries in psychiatry,* London, 1967. With reviews of the literature and bibliographies. With a complete bibliography of the author's publications, 1926-1966.] London, Routledge & Paul, 1967; N.Y., Science House, 1968, © 1967. 310 pp. Pp. 235-252.

The Paul H. Hoch Award Lecture. American Psychopathological Association.

1st. 1967. Wootton, Barbara, Baroness Wootton of Abinger. Social psychiatry and psychopathology; a layman's comments on contemporary development. *In* Zubin, Joseph, and Freyhan, Fritz Adolf, eds. *Social psychiatry;* the proceedings of the Fifty-seventh Annual Meeting of the American Psychopathological Association, held in New York City, February 1967. [With an introductory sketch: Lady Wootton of Abinger, Paul H. Hoch award lecturer, 1967, by Sir Aubrey Lewis. With the Paul H. Hoch award lecture for 1967: Social psychiatry and psychopathology: a layman's comments on contemporary developments, by Barbara Wootton (Lady Wootton of Abinger). With the presidential address by Bernard C. Glueck, Jr.: Automation and social change. With reviews of the literature and bibliographies.] N.Y., Grune & Stratton; London, Heinemann Medical Books [distributor], 1968. 382 pp. Pp. 283-299.

Hunterian Orations. Royal College of Surgeons of England, London.

1872. Jackson, John Hughlings. The physiological aspects of education. [Abstract.] *In* Jackson, John Hughlings. *Selected writings.* Ed. for the guarantors of "Brain" by James Taylor, with the advice and assistance of Gordon Holmes and F. M. R. Walshe. 1st ed., 1931, reprinted. N.Y., Basic Books, 1958; London, Staples Press, 1959. 2 v. Vol. 2. Pp. 265-269.

Alexander James Inglis Lectureship in Secondary Education. Harvard University.

1954. Smith, Henry Lee. *Linguistic science and the teaching of English.* Cambridge, Harvard Univ. Pr., 1956. 61 pp. (The Inglis lecture, 1954.)

Hughlings Jackson Lecture. Neurological Society, London.

1st. 1897. Jackson, John Hughlings. Relations of different divisions of the central nervous system to one another and to parts of the body. *In* Jackson, John Hughlings. *Selected writings.* Ed. for the guarantors of "Brain" by James Taylor, with the advice and assistance of Gordon Holmes and F. M. R. Walshe. 1st ed., 1931, reprinted. N.Y., Basic Books, 1958; London, Staples Press, 1959. 2 v. Vol. 2. Pp. 422-443.

The Kappa Delta Pi Lecture Series.

Vol. 35. 1963. Maslow, Abraham Harold. *Religions, values, and peak-experiences.* [Series editor's introd. by E. I. F. Williams. With a bibliography.] Columbus, Ohio State Univ. Pr., 1964. 123 pp. (The Kappa Delta Pi lecture series, vol. 35.)

The Herbert Sidney Langfeld Memorial Lectures. Department of Psychology, Princeton University.

1st. 1965. Von Békésy, Georg. *Sensory inhibition.* [Outgrowth of the author's experiments carried out from 1927 to the present, in the Hungarian Institute for Research in Telegraphy and in the Physical Institute of the University in Budapest, in the Royal Institute of Technology in Stockholm, at Harvard University, and in hospitals and doctors' offices. Edited by E. G. Wever. The first Herbert Sidney Langfeld memorial lectures, delivered 1965 in the Department of Psychology, Princeton University. With a prefatory statement by the Herbert Sidney Langfeld Memorial Lecture Committee, F. A. Geldard, chairman. With a list of the author's publications, 1928-1966, and a bibliography.] Princeton, N.J., Princeton Univ. Pr.; London, Oxford Univ. Pr. [distributor], 1967. 265 pp. (The Herbert Sidney Langfeld memorial lectures, 1965.)

The Florina Lasker Lectures. New York School of Social Work, Columbia University.

2nd. 1953. Myrdal, Alva Reiner, Altmeyer, Arthur J., and Rusk, Dean. *America's role in international social science.* N.Y., Columbia Univ. Pr., 1955. 109 pp. (The Florina Lasker lectures, 1953.)

Lumleian Lectures. Royal College of Physicians of London.

1890. Jackson, John Hughlings. On convulsive seizures. *In* Jackson, John Hughlings. *Selected writings.* Ed. for the guarantors of "Brain" by James Taylor, with the advice and assistance of Gordon Holmes and F. M. R. Walshe. 1st ed., 1931, reprinted. N.Y., Basic Books, 1958; London, Staples Press, 1959. 2 v. Vol. 1. Pp. 412-423.

The MacIver Lectureship. American Sociological Association.

1962. Goffman, Erving. *Stigma; notes on the management of spoiled identity.* [Presented in an earlier version as the MacIver Lecture at the Southern Sociological Society, Louisville, Kentucky, April 13, 1962.] Englewood Cliffs, N.J., London, Prentice-Hall, 1963. 147 pp. (A Spectrum book, S-73.)

J. S. Manson Lectures. Royal Institute of Philosophy, London.

2nd. 1948. Lewis, Sir Aubrey Julian. Philosophy and psychiatry. *In* Lewis, Sir Aubrey Julian. *The state of psychiatry: essays and addresses* [previously published, 1934-1965. Edited by the author's students to mark his retirement from the Maudsley Hospital in 1966. Companion volume to the author's *Inquiries in psychiatry,* London, 1967. With reviews of the literature and bibliographies. With a complete bibliography of the author's publications, 1926-1966.] London, Routledge & Paul, 1967; N.Y., Science House, 1968, © 1967. 310 pp. Pp. 163-194.

W. M. Martin Lectures. College of Law, University of Saskatchewan.

1962. Hartung, Frank E. *Crime, law and society.* [Based on the W. M. Martin lectures for 1962, College of Law, University of Saskatchewan. With a bibliography.] Detroit, Wayne State Univ. Pr., 1965. 320 pp. Paperback ed.: Detroit, Wayne State Univ. Pr., 1966. 320 pp. (Waynebook, WB 21.)

Josiah Mason Lectures in Anthropology. University of Birmingham.

1953. Sprott, Walter John Herbert. *Science and social action.* Josiah Mason lectures delivered at the University of Birmingham. Glencoe, Ill., Free Press; London, Watts, 1954. 164 pp. (Birmingham, Eng. University. Josiah Mason lectures in anthropology, 1953.)

Ballard Matthews Lectures. University College of North Wales, Bangor.

1960. Mather, Kenneth. *Human diversity; the nature and significance of differences among men.* [Based on the Ballard Matthews lectures given at the University College of North Wales, 1960. With a bibliography.] N.Y., Free Press; Edinburgh, Oliver & Boyd, 1964. 126 pp.

Maudsley Lectures. Royal Medico-Psychological Association, London.

25th. 1950. Lewis, Sir Aubrey Julian. Henry Maudsley: his work and influence. *In* Lewis, Sir Aubrey Julian. *The state of psychiatry: essays and addresses* [previously published, 1934-1965. Edited by the author's students to mark his retirement from the Maudsley Hospital in 1966. Companion volume to the author's *Inquiries in psychiatry,* London, 1967. With reviews of the literature and bibliographies. With a complete bibliography of the author's publications, 1926-1966.] London, Routledge & Paul, 1967; N.Y., Science House, 1968, © 1967. 310 pp. Pp. 29-48.

The A. W. Mellon Lectures in the Fine Arts. National Gallery of Art, Washington, D.C.

5th. 1956. Gombrich, Ernst Hans Josef. *Art and illusion; a study in the psychology of pictorial representation.* N.Y., Pantheon Books; London, Phaidon Press, 1960. 466 pp. (Bollingen series, 35, 5. The A. W. Mellon lectures in the fine arts, 1956) New ed. reset: London, Phaidon Press, 1962. 388 pp.

The Adolf Meyer Research Lecture. American Psychiatric Association.

1960. Lewis, Sir Aubrey Julian. The study of defect. *In* Lewis, Sir Aubrey Julian. *The state of psychiatry: essays and addresses* [previously published, 1934-1965. Edited by the author's students to mark his retirement from the Maudsley Hospital in 1966. Companion volume to the author's *Inquiries in psychiatry,* London, 1967. With reviews of the literature and bibliographies. With a complete bibliography of the author's publications, 1926-1966.] London, Routledge & Paul, 1967; N.Y., Science House, 1968, © 1967. 310 pp. Pp. 214-234.

The Lucile P. Morrison Lectures. Western Behavioral Sciences Institute, La Jolla, California.

1961-1964. The Lucile P. Morrison Lectures. *In* Farson, Richard Evans, ed. *Science and human affairs.* [Twelve of the sixteen Lucile P. Morrison lectures given 1961-1964 under the sponsorship of the Western Behavioral Sciences Institute. Authors: Gardner Murphy and others. Edited

and with an introd.: Can science solve human dilemmas? by Richard E. Farson. With bibliographies.] Palo Alto, Calif., Science and Behavior Books, 1965. 214 pp.
Murphy, Gardner. Where is the human race going? *ibid.*, pp. 7-17.
Rogers, Carl Ransom. A humanistic conception of man. *ibid.*, pp. 18-31.
Huxley, Aldous Leonard. Human potentialities. *ibid.*, pp. 32-44.
Maslow, Abraham Harold. Lessons from the peak experiences. *ibid.*, pp. 45-54.
Koch, Sigmund. The allures of ameaning in modern psychology. *ibid.*, pp. 55-82.
Newcomb, Theodore Mead. Aspects of the acquaintance process. *ibid.*, pp. 83-94.
Hayakawa, Samuel Ichiyé. The use and misuse of language; some thoughts on communication with one's children. *ibid.*, pp. 95-113.
Hilgard, Ernest Ropiequet. Developmental-interactive aspects of hypnosis. *ibid.*, pp. 114-126.
Gerard, Ralph Waldo. Memory; fixation of experience. *ibid.*, pp. 127-139.
Allport, Gordon Willard. Prejudice in perspective. *ibid.*, pp. 140-149.
Osgood, Charles Egerton. An alternative to war or surrender. *ibid.*, pp. 150-165.
Kelman, Herbert C. From dystopia to utopia; an analysis of Huxley's *Island*. *ibid.*, pp. 166-184.
Taylor, Harold. Science and art. *ibid.*, pp. 185-196.
Gibb, Jack R. Fear and facade. *ibid.*, pp. 197-214.

Munro Lectures. University of Edinburgh.

1953. Clark, Sir Wilfrid Edward Le Gros. *The antecedents of man; an introduction to the evolution of the primates.* [Originally delivered as the 1953 Munro lectures at the University of Edinburgh under the title, The paleontology of the primates and the problem of human ancestry.] Edinburgh, Edinburgh Univ. Pr., 1959. 374 pp. (Edinburgh. University. Publications: science and mathematics, 2) Chicago, Quadrangle Books, 1960, © 1959. 374 pp.

1966. Banton, Michael Parker. *Race relations.* [Based in part on the author's Munro lectures for 1966, delivered at the University of Edinburgh, and on his previous publications, 1959-1963. With a survey of racial thought before Darwin. With reviews of the literature and a bibliography.] London, Tavistock, 1967; N.Y., Basic Books, © 1967. 434 pp.

National Children's Home Convocation Lecture. National Children's Home, London.

1959. Wall, William Douglas. *Child of our times; cultural change and the challenge to healthy mental growth.* London, National Children's Home, 1959. 110 pp. (National Children's Home convocation lecture, 1959.)

The George B. Pegram Lectures. Brookhaven National Laboratory.

2nd. 1960. Dubos, René Jules. *The dreams of reason; science and utopias.* [Based on the second George B. Pegram lectures, delivered at the Brookhaven National Laboratory in October, 1960. Prefatory statement: The George B. Pegram lectures, by Gerhart Friedlander, Samuel A. Goudsmit, Leland J. Haworth, Daniel E. Koshland, Jr., James S. Robertson, and R. Christian Anderson, chairman.] N.Y., London, Columbia Univ. Pr., 1961. 167 pp. (The George B. Pegram lectures.)

Anson G. Phelps Lectureship on Early American History. James Stokes Foundation, New York University.

1959. Shryock, Richard Harrison. *Medicine and society in America, 1660-1860.* N.Y., New York Univ. Pr., 1960. 182 pp. (Anson G. Phelps lectureship on early American history, 1959.)

Porter Lectures. University of Kansas School of Medicine.

Ser. 22. Kubie, Lawrence Schlesinger. *Neurotic distortion of the creative process.* Lawrence, Univ. of Kansas Pr., 1958. 151 pp. (Kansas. University. School of Medicine. Porter lectures, ser. 22.)

The Isaac Ray Award Lectures. American Psychiatric Association.

1st. 1952. Overholser, Winfred. *The psychiatrist and the law.* N.Y., Harcourt, Brace, 1953. 147 pp. (The Isaac Ray award book.)

2nd. 1953. Zilboorg, Gregory. *The psychology of the criminal act and punishment.* N.Y., Harcourt, Brace, 1954. 141 pp. (The Isaac Ray award series) London, Hogarth Press, 1954. 141 pp. (Psycho-analytical epitomes, no. 5.)

3rd. 1954. Biggs, John. *The guilty mind.* N.Y., Harcourt, Brace, 1955. 236 pp. (The Isaac Ray award series) Paperback ed.: Baltimore, Johns Hopkins Press; London, Oxford Univ. Pr. [distributor], 1967. 236 pp.

4th. 1955. Weihofen, Henry. *The urge to punish; new approaches to the problem of mental irresponsibility for crime.* N.Y., Farrar, Straus & Cudahy, 1956. 213 pp. (Isaac Ray award book) British ed.: With a foreword by Lord Russell of Liverpool. London, Gollancz, 1957. 213 pp. (Isaac Ray lectures, 1955.)

5th. 1957. Roche, Philip Quintin. *The criminal mind; a study of communication between the criminal law and psychiatry.* N.Y., Farrar, Straus & Cudahy, 1958. 299 pp. N.Y., Grove Press, 1959. 299 pp. (Evergreen book E-176.)

1962. Glueck, Sheldon. *Law and psychiatry: cold war or entente cordiale?* Baltimore, Johns Hopkins Press, 1962; London, Tavistock, 1963.181 pp. (The Isaac Ray award lectures, 1962) Paperback ed.: Baltimore, Johns Hopkins Press, 1966. 181 pp. (JH17.)

1963, 1964, 1966. Menninger, Karl Augustus. *The crime of punishment* [An expansion of the author's Isaac Ray award lectures given at Columbia University December 5, 1963, and April 14, 1964, and at the University of Kansas April 14, 1966, as a part of its Centennial Anniversary.] The Isaac Ray award book. [Dedicated to Jeanetta Lyle Menninger. With case illustrations and bibliographies.] N.Y., Viking Press, 1968. 305 pp. (The Isaac Ray award lectures, 1963, 1964, 1966.)

1966. Stürup, Georg Kristoffer. *Treating the "untreatable"; chronic criminals at Herstedvester.* [An account of the work done in the Herstedvester Detention Centre at Albertslund, Denmark, since the author became its superintendent in 1942. Based on the Isaac Ray award lectures prepared for the Isaac Ray award of the American Psychiatric Association for 1966, expanded into book form during the author's stay as a visiting scholar at the Center for Studies in Criminal Justice of the University of Chicago Law School. With extensive case histories.] Baltimore, Johns Hopkins Press; London, Oxford Univ. Pr. [distributor], 1968. 266 pp. (The Isaac Ray award lectures, 1966.)

The Rede Lecture. Cambridge University.

1959. Snow, Sir Charles Percy. *The two cultures and the scientific revolution.* N.Y., Columbia Univ. Pr.; London, Cambridge Univ. Pr., 1959. 58 pp. (American ed.); 51 pp. (British ed.) (The Rede lecture, 1959.)

Mary Hemingway Rees Memorial Lectures on Mental Health and Spiritual Values. World Federation for Mental Health, London.

2nd. 1960. Baruk, Henri. *Hebraic civilization and the science of man.* Transl. from the French by Philip Polack. [Foreword by E. E. Krapf. With a bibliography.] N.Y., London, World Federation for Mental Health, 1961. 75 pp. (Mary Hemingway Rees memorial lecture, 2d, 1960.) (A World Mental Health Year publication.)

The BBC Reith Lectures. British Broadcasting Corporation, London.

1959. Medawar, Peter Brian. *The future of man.* N.Y., Basic Books; London, Methuen, 1960, © 1959. 128 pp. (The BBC Reith lectures, 1959.)

1962. Carstairs, George Morris. *This island now; the surge of social change in the twentieth century.* [With an introd. including passages from an article on the Reith lectures first published in The Scotsman on 24th December 1962 and with bibliographies.] N.Y., Basic Books, © 1962. 102 pp. (The B.B.C. Reith lectures, 1962.) British ed.: *This island now.* London, Hogarth Press, 1963, © 1962. 102 pp. (The B.B.C. Reith lectures, 1962.)

Riddell Memorial Lectures. University of Durham.

30th ser. 1958. Brain, Sir Walter Russell. *The nature of experience.* N.Y. London, Oxford Univ. Pr., 1959. 73 pp.

(Riddell memorial lectures [Durham University, Durham, Eng.] 30th ser., 1958.)

Bertram H. Roberts Memorial Lectures. Yale University.

4th. 1960. Lewis, Sir Aubrey Julian. Ebb and flow in social psychiatry. *In* Lewis, Sir Aubrey Julian. *The state of psychiatry: essays and addresses* [previously published 1934-1965. Edited by the author's students to mark his retirement from the Maudsley Hospital in 1966. Companion volume to the author's *Inquiries in psychiatry,* London, 1967. With reviews of the literature and bibliographies. With a complete bibliography of the author's publications, 1926-1966.] London, Routledge & Paul, 1967; N.Y., Science House, 1968, ©1967. 310 pp. Pp. 253-272.

The Charles Russell Memorial Lecture. Trustees: The Head of the Children's Department of the Home Office; the General Secretary, the National Association of Boys' Clubs, London.

11th. 1963. Walker, Nigel. *Adolescent maladjustment.* London, 1963. 15 pp. (Charles Russell memorial lecture, 11th.) (Purchase from The Trustees, Charles Russell Memorial Lecture, 17 Bedford Square, London, W.C. 1.)

The Thomas William Salmon Memorial Lectures. New York Academy of Medicine.

1st. 1932. Meyer, Adolf. *Psychobiology; a science of man.* With a foreword by Nolan D. C. Lewis. Comp. and ed. by Eunice E. Winters and Anna Mae Bowers. Springfield, Ill., Thomas; Oxford, Blackwell, 1957. 257 pp. (The Thomas William Salmon memorial lectures.)

1952. Kallmann, Franz Josef. *Heredity in health and mental disorder; principles of psychiatric genetics in the light of comparative twin studies.* With a foreword by Nolan D. C. Lewis. N.Y. Norton, 1953. 315 pp. (The Thomas William Salmon memorial lectures.)

1953. Linton, Ralph. *Culture and mental disorders.* Ed. by George Devereux. Springfield, Ill., Thomas; Oxford, Blackwell, 1956. 139 pp.

1956. Magoun, Horace Winchell. *The waking brain.* Springfield, Ill., Thomas; Oxford, Blackwell, 1958. 138 pp. (The Thomas William Salmon memorial lecture.)

1958. Leighton, Alexander Hamilton. *An introduction to social psychiatry.* Springfield, Ill., Thomas; Oxford, Blackwell, 1960. 110 pp. (The Thomas William Salmon memorial lectures.)

1964. Farnsworth, Dana Lyda. *Psychiatry, education, and the young adult.* [A discussion of the role of psychiatry in colleges and universities.] With a foreword by Francis J. Braceland. [With case histories and bibliographies.] Springfield, Ill., Thomas, 1966. 268 pp. (The Thomas William Salmon memorial lectures.)

Mona Bronfman Sheckman Lectures in Social Psychiatry. Tulane University.

1961. Lidz, Theodore. *The family and human adaptation; three lectures* [presented at Tulane University, February 23 and 24, 1961. Based on studies of families with schizophrenic offspring.] N.Y., International Universities Press, 1963. 120 pp. (Mona Bronfman Sheckman lectures in social psychiatry, 1961.) London, Hogarth Press, 1964. 120 pp. (Mona Bronfman Sheckman lectures in social psychiatry, 1961.) (International psychoanalytical library, no. 60.)

Mrs. Hepsa Ely Silliman Memorial Lectures. Yale University.

no date. Granit, Ragnar. *Receptors and sensory perception; a discussion of aims, means, and results of electrophysiological research into the process of reception.* New Haven, Yale Univ. Pr.; London, Oxford Univ. Pr., 1955. 369 pp. (Yale University, Mrs. Hepsa Ely Silliman memorial lectures.)

no date. Spence, Kenneth Wartenbee. *Behavior theory and conditioning.* New Haven, Yale Univ. Pr.; London, Oxford Univ. Pr., 1956. 262 pp. (Yale University, Mrs. Hepsa Ely Silliman memorial lectures.)

1959. Vol. 38. Dobzhansky, Theodosius Grigorievich. *Mankind evolving; the evolution of the human species.* New Haven, Conn., London, Yale Univ. Pr., 1962. 381 pp. (Yale University. Mrs. Hepsa Ely Silliman memorial lectures, 1959.)

The Watson Smith Lecture. Royal College of Physicians of London.

1966. Sargant, William Walters. Psychiatric treatment in general teaching hospitals: a plea for a mechanistic approach. *In* Sargant, William Walters. *The unquiet mind; the autobiography of a physician in psychological medicine.* [Prepared for publication in collaboration with Robert Graves.] With a pref. by D. Ewen Cameron. [With an appendix: Psychiatric treatment in general teaching hospitals: a plea for a mechanistic approach: the Watson Smith lecture given by the author at the Royal College of Physicians, reprinted from the *British Medical Journal,* 1966, 2, 257-262. With a bibliography.] Boston, Little, Brown, 1967. 240 pp. (An Atlantic Monthly press book.) London, Heinemann, 1967. 240 pp. Pp. 217-230.

Dwight Harrington Terry Foundation Lectures on Religion in the Light of Science and Philosophy. Yale University.

1954. Allport, Gordon Willard. *Becoming; basic considerations for a psychology of personality.* New Haven, Yale Univ. Pr., 1955. 106 pp. (The Terry lectures) London, Oxford Univ. Pr., 1955. Paperback ed.: New Haven, Conn., Yale Univ. Pr.; London, Oxford Univ. Pr., 1960. 106 pp.

1963. Vol. 34. Mead, Margaret. *Continuities in cultural evolution.* [With bibliographies.] New Haven, Conn., London, Yale Univ. Pr., 1964. 471 pp. (The Dwight Harrington Terry Foundation lectures on religion in the light of science and philosophy, Yale University, vol. 34.)

Vanuxem Lectures. Louis Clark Vanuxem Foundation. Princeton University.

1956. Penfield, Wilder, & Roberts, Lamar. *Speech and brain-mechanisms.* Based on the Vanuxem lectures given by Wilder Penfield at Princeton University in February, 1956. Princeton, N.J., Princeton Univ. Pr.: London, Oxford Univ. Pr., 1959. 286 pp.

Charles R. Walgreen Foundation Lectures. Charles R. Walgreen Foundation for the Study of American Institutions. University of Chicago.

1956. Arendt, Hannah. *The human condition.* Chicago, Univ. of Chicago Pr.; London, Cambridge Univ. Pr., 1958. 332 pp. (Charles R. Walgreen Foundation lectures.)

Heinz Werner Lecture Series in Developmental Psychology and Related Disciplines. Heinz Werner Institute of Developmental Psychology, Clark University.

1st. 1966. Bertalanffy, Ludwig von. *Organismic psychology and systems theory.* [Two lectures, "The organismic concept in psychology and biology," and "The open system of science—toward a new 'natural philosophy,' " representing the first in the Heinz Werner Lecture Series in Developmental Psychology and Related Disciplines, 1966, sponsored by the Heinz Werner Institute of Developmental Psychology, Clark University. With a pref.: The Heinz Werner lecture series, by Bernard Kaplan, Seymour Wapner, and Joachim F. Wohlwill. Foreword by Howard B. Jefferson. With a bibliography.] Worcester, Mass., Clark Univ. Pr. with Barre Publishers, 1968. 76 pp. (Heinz Werner lectures, 1966.)

Bertalanffy, Ludwig von. *Robots, men, and minds: psychology in the modern world.* [Based upon the Heinz Werner inaugural lectures presented by the author at Clark University, January 13 and 14, 1966. With a bibliography.] N.Y., Braziller, 1967. 150 pp.

2nd. 1967. Piaget, Jean. *On the development of memory and identity.* [Two lectures, "Memory and operations of intelligence," based on a book then in press with title *Mémoire et intelligence* by J. Piaget and B. Inhelder in collaboration with H. Sinclair, Paris, 1968, and Identity and conservation, based on a volume of *Études d'épistémologie génétique,* Paris, 1968.] Translated by Eleanor Duckworth. [With a pref.: The Heinz Werner lecture series, by Bernard Kaplan, Seymour Wapner, and Joachim F. Wohlwill. The second volume in the lecture series, sponsored by the Heinz Werner Institute of Developmental Psychology, Clark University. With a bibliography.] Worcester, Mass., Clark Univ. Pr. with

Barre Publishers, 1968. 42 pp. (Heinz Werner lectures, 1967.)

William Alanson White Memorial Lectures. William Alanson White Psychiatric Foundation.

1st. 1939. Sullivan, Harry Stack. *Conceptions of modern psychiatry.* With a foreword by the author and a critical appraisal of the theory by Patrick Mullahy. 2d ed. with a pref. by Dexter M. Bullard. London, Tavistock, 1955. 298 pp. (William Alanson White memorial lectures, 1st.)

William Withering Memorial Lectureship. University of Birmingham.

1960. Young, John Zachary. *A model of the brain.* [Based upon] the William Withering lectures delivered to the Faculty of Medicine of the University of Birmingham 1960 with the title: Mechanisms of learning and form discrimination. N.Y., Oxford Univ. Pr.; Oxford, Clarendon Press, 1964. 348 pp.

# ESSAY 13

## *The Developmental Sciences: A Bibliographic Analysis of a Trend*

Originally published as Editorial in *Mental Health Book Review Index*, vol. 16 (whole no. 21), 1971.

### WHAT ARE THE DEVELOPMENTAL SCIENCES?

Development in nature and in the condition and affairs of man has never been as intensively studied as it is today. A worldwide effort is now under way to bring this work into focus and to utilize its fruits for the betterment of human life. This process has not been heralded, however, as was the advent of the behavioral sciences. In the mid-1950's that term began to make its way from being a semantic puzzle to becoming a household word, as familiar to the educated public and to policy makers as to the scientific community. A decade later the less artificial, if no less elusive, term "developmental sciences" entered the behavioral science literature as if it were self-explanatory and without arousing any discussion.

The term "developmental sciences" as currently used provides a unifying name for work in the behavioral sciences that results from, and contributes to, theory and research concerning the growth and development of man and animals. At the core of the developmental sciences is developmental psychology, the first specialty to be so designated. In 1967, a contributor to the symposium, *The Neuropsychology of Development*, characterized this field in words that capture the spirit of the new trend: "Although one could easily form a different impression from the number of texts and articles on the subject, *developmental psychology* represents an approach to problems rather than a distinct subject matter. Almost any psychological problem can be approached developmentally. . . ." He then set forth the advantages that result from asking how a particular phenomenon came about and from considering the nature of the changes that occur in organisms as they interact with the environment (Ref. 1, p. 1). These observations are also true for the developmental sciences in the broader sense suggested here.

A relationship between the developmental and the behavioral sciences was first implied when the Developmental Sciences Trust, founded in England in 1967 under the chairmanship of Lord Adrian, made known its plan to open a "Centre for Advanced Study in the Developmental Sciences," a name obviously modeled after that of the influential Center for Advanced Study in the Behavioral Sciences at Palo Alto, California. The first two volumes of proceedings of international study groups held under the joint auspices of the projected Centre and the Ciba Foundation, 1967 and 1968, in a program on "The Origins of Human Behavior," described the Centre's activities as related "to all those sciences and disciplines that can contribute to greater knowledge of the biological, social and psychological principles that govern the development and functioning of human behavior over the life-cycle." In addition to stimulating and co-ordinating research and fostering a developmental perspective on human nature, the Centre was "to encourage the application of knowledge from the developmental sciences by those, in all sectors of society, engaged in coping with or preventing human problems."[2,3] Although, according to information obtained from the Ciba Foundation, the project of opening the Centre has since been abandoned, the Developmental Sciences Trust continues to organize international study groups and to pursue the initial scientific aim.

In 1968, the article on "developmental psychology" in the *International Encyclopedia of the Social Sciences* referred to the National Institute of Child Health and Human Development (NICHD) as established "to provide leadership in training of investigators and research in developmental sciences including developmental psychology." There was no further explanation. Since 1963, when NICHD was founded as one of the National Institutes of Health, the annual reports of the Depart-

## THE CONCEPT OF DEVELOPMENT

Definitions of development relating to a general theory, apart from concrete applications, are hard to find, with one notable exception. Contributors to a Conference on the Concept of Development, held in 1955 at the University of Minnesota,[4] addressed themselves to this question. They pointed out the variety of meanings of the word "development." It can be used to connote a process or the product of a process. If interpreted in the original sense of the word as an unfolding, development means a sequence of continuous changes, leading to an outcome that is potentially present in the earlier stages of the process. In contemporary theory, the older "preformistic" ideas have been replaced by an "epigenetic" view, which acknowledges that organization is created anew in development. Not every sequence of changes is designated as developmental. The changes must be cumulative and irreversible and, in addition, they must lead to a new mode of organization in the developing system, with an increased capacity for self-regulation and independence. The construct of "directiveness" is implied in the definition of organic development in its two major aspects, namely, that the developmental process involves progressive changes from a more simple to a more complex organization, and that development proceeds from the general to the specific. One of the contributors to this 1955 Conference, Heinz Werner, combined these two aspects into one regulative principle of development, "which states that wherever development occurs it proceeds from a state of relative globality and lack of differentiation to a state of increasing differentiation, articulation, and hierarchic integration." He also discussed development not only in the light of specific theories and principles but "as a concept that proposes a certain manner of viewing behavior in its manifold manifestations." He recognized, therefore, the potentially unifying influence on the life sciences of the developmental approach, with its basic assumption "that wherever there is life there is growth and development, that is, formation in terms of systematic, orderly sequence." In analogy to a unified developmental biology, Werner saw developmental psychology as providing a single framework for forms of behavior observed in such varied fields as comparative animal psychology, child psychology, psychopathology, ethnopsychology, and the psychology of man in our own culture (Ref. 4, pp. 125-126).

# THE WORD "DEVELOPMENT" IN RECENT BOOK TITLES

Present bibliographic techniques and systems do not identify work concerned with developmental theory, research, and methodology, in a form that would permit observing the progress of the developmental sciences. Publications recording this work remain embedded in the literature of the behavioral sciences and the various parent disciplines, which are as diverse and separately organized as genetics, neurology, ethology, psychology, gerontology, and education, to name a few of the many contributory fields.

Books that use the word development, or a close variant, in the title or subtitle, may provide first clues for identifying developmental studies. The present sample contains more than fifty such books. They vary greatly, however, especially with respect to their scope and the developmental processes specified as the object of study. A number of these books are compendia by one or more authors, or reviews of progress. Notable among these are Baldwin's *Theories of Child Development,* Hoffman and Hoffman's *Review of Child Development Research, Advances in Child Development and Behavior,* Brackbill's *Infancy and Early Childhood: a Handbook and Guide to Human Development,* and *Annual Progress in Child Psychiatry and Child Development.*[5-9] The emphasis on child development in these titles is striking. Two other books concerned with developmental theories and concepts are equally limited.[10-11] One historical treatment is more comprehensive,[12] one presentation of an author's "epigenetic view" is based on his animal studies.[13]

In many of the books the term "development" appears in a specific context, for example, development in learning, cognition, perception,[14-18] development of the brain and of sex differences,[19-21] of role-taking and communication skills and political attitudes,[22-23] character, conscience, and moral development.[24-26] Three titles lead to Piaget,[27-29] four to the approaches of comparative and psychoanalytic psychology, psychobiology, and neuropsychology.[30-32,1] Other books are concerned with the psychopathology of mental development or, more specifically, with studies of language disability and of babies with mongolism,[33-36] a few with giving therapeutic help in developing ego and ego-social functions and other cases of developmental problems.[37-39] Personality development appears as a topic by itself and in diverse contexts such as social class and race, marriage, death in the family, and play therapy.[40-44] Finally, the term is used in relation to obvious developmental stages: infancy, preadolescence, and the whole life cycle.[45-48]

Two of the titles refer to community and political development.[49-50] "Development" as used in economics, sociology, political science, and other social sciences is not, however, now encompassed by developmental research, which is limited to the study of living organisms. The remaining titles in the sample use "development" in the sense of advances in theory or research in a special field. They are mentioned here only as a reminder that "development" as a technical term has to be clearly established. This should not be more difficult, however, than it was in the 1950's to establish the difference between "child behavior" and the good or bad behavior of a child.

## DEVELOPMENTAL STAGES AND THE LIFE CYCLE

Further clues to current trends in the developmental sciences may be found in books explicitly concerned with major developmental stages, with what one contributor to the 1955 Conference on the Concept of Development called "the age-bound behavior of the person as it takes on form or shape . . . the person whom we study from birth on to maturity" (Ref. 4, p. 25). Ideas about the periods encompassed in the life cycle have been changing, especially in recent decades, and this central aspect of the developmental sciences is even now far from crystallized. Not only have the major stages become more closely subdivided, as more and more transitional periods have been recognized and studied, but the concept of the life cycle as a whole has been extended at both ends.

As early as 1911, Baldwin's *Dictionary of Philosophy and Psychology* defined (biological) "development" as "the entire series of vital changes normal to the individual organism, from its origin from the parent cell or cells until death." This inclusive meaning was lost sight of during the period of progressing research, which only now, six decades later, has caught up with the earlier formulation. To embryology, one of the oldest and primary disciplines in the province of the developmental sciences, more recent multidisciplinary studies of prenatal and perinatal influences on development have been added. A further extension in this direction may come about if "genetic engineering" and related work aimed at changing the hereditary basis of life, which is as yet only on the horizon, should become a scientific and social reality. At the other end, studies of aging and the aged have been drawn together in the still relatively young, multidisciplinary field of gerontology. A further extension, which makes the study of death and dying germane to the developmental sciences, is becoming manifest right now. This may account in part for the dramatic increase in the recent literature related to death. Theodore Lidz has made the point explicit: "It may seem strange for an unconsidered moment to conclude this guide to the life cycle with a chapter on death. But death is part of the life cycle, an inevitable outcome of life that brings closure to a life story; and, because the human from early childhood is aware of his ultimate death, it influences his development and his way of life profoundly" (Ref. 48, p. 496).

Even when, as before, only the titles of books are considered, the present limited sample of the literature of the developmental sciences covers all the stages of the life span. Joffe[51] reviews research "which relates events prior to birth to effects on the postnatal behavior of organisms." *Childbearing,* a volume of critical reviews of studies of reproduction with a social-science viewpoint,[52] grew out of the rising concern about the social aspects of developmental stages that had long been approached only from a biomedical point of view. Other trends are illustrated in three books on infancy: interest in data from non-Western cultures;[53] a historical interest, shown in a collection of readings going back to 1907;[54] and the search for an understanding of normal development, the subject of Escalona's study.[46]

Escalona's research spans the period from the mid-1940's to the mid-1960's and thus coincides with the formative period of the developmental sciences in the current sense. Her introductory review of trends in research, which shows the fluctuations of interest in the neonate and earliest infancy, contributes to an understanding of the difference between the vast field of child study and developmental science. Interest in the extensive studies of newborns carried out during the 1920's and 1930's waned because they were purely descriptive and not effectively linked to a developmental theory. In contrast, the researchers of more recent years have been concerned with the implications of their work for the study of human development. They have, for example, focused their interest on factors that co-determine the course of subsequent development, on the processes and mechanisms that constitute developmental change, and on determining what continuity exists between learning processes during the early months of life and learning processes at later ages (Ref. 46, pp. 3-6).

Data that potentially lend themselves to longitudinal studies can, therefore, become an important resource for the developmental sciences. Perhaps the most comprehensive longitudinal research yet undertaken resulted from the study of 17,000 babies born during one week in March 1958 in England, Scotland, and Wales, which had then yielded perinatal data said to be unparalleled in the world. Another part of this project, conducted in the mid-1960's, forms the first report of the National Child Development Study, *11,000 Seven-Year-Olds.*[55] More typical of longitudinal development research, however, are intensive studies of relatively small samples, for example, in Escalona's book, the 32 infants selected from the 128 studied in her previous project entitled *Early Phases of Personality Development,* and the 42 children selected from the 136 in the longitudinal study begun by Thomas and others in 1956.[56] The importance of such data for developmental research is underlined by the interlocking of projects. For instance, the authors of *Personality Development at Preadolescence*—in part an outgrowth of the Longitudinal Study Project at the Menninger Foundation—drew their subjects, sixty boys and girls 9 to 13 years old, from the group of children from the Topeka, Kansas, area studied in infancy by Escalona.[47]

## THE LIFE CYCLE AFTER CHILDHOOD

Some of the studies on adolescence have resulted from projects conducted over periods of four or five years: the Symptomatic Adolescent Research Project reported in *The Psychiatric Dilemma of Adolescence,*[57] and the Modal Adolescent Project, which Offer reported in his book subtitled *A Study of Normal Adolescent Boys.*[58] In addition to Offer's study, a report issued by the Group for the Advancement of Psychiatry, *Normal Adolescence,*[59] shows that psychiatrists share the psychologists' interest in normal development. The next phase of the trend relates the study of problems of adolescence to psychosocial and sociocultural forces. Examples are two volumes resulting from international congresses, one concerned broadly with psychosocial perspectives, the other specifically with adolescent drug dependence,[60-61] a British study of *The Sexual Behaviour of Young People,*[62] and *Minority Group Adolescents in the United States,* a collection of papers concerning Negro, Mexican, Puerto Rican, Oriental, and American Indian adolescents, introduced with an essay, "Adolescents as a United States Minority Group in an Era of Social Change."[63]

Two books on postadolescence and the young adult present aspects of psychotherapy,[64-65] but one resulting from a social Psychology Symposium again pursues the social theme, as indicated in the title: *Problems of Youth: Transition to Adulthood in a Changing World.*[66]

A beginning toward filling a gap in the literature on the developmental stages, the study of middle life, was made when the Scientific Committee of the World Federation for Mental Health initiated a survey of research relating to the 40-60 age period and then discussed the data.[67] Another effort to bring together the literature on middle age and aging took the form of a reader in social psychology, based mainly on publications of the period 1956-1968.[68] Research conducted in England in the early 1960's with 90 persons in the age range from 20 to 79 is reported in *Age and Function* by Heron and Chown, assisted by the Staff of the Medical Research Council Unit for Research on Occupational Aspects of Aging.[69]

Some of the books on aging reflect the thinking that has brought gerontology into the mainstream of the developmental sciences. In the preface to his *The Psychology of Human Ageing,*[70] Bromley observes: "We spend about one quarter of our lives growing up and three quarters growing old." He considers the study of human aging a logical extension of developmental psychology, and finds it strange "that psychologists and others have devoted most of their efforts to the study of childhood and adolescence." The foreword to this book by B. M. Foss notes, however, "that psychologists have already come to regard the study of old age as part of developmental psychology, with the implication that development never stops." This comment carries special weight in view of the fact that its author is the Executive Chairman of the Developmental Sciences Trust mentioned at the beginning of this essay. The editor of a series of studies representing recent advances in research and theory on human aging relates the notable growth of this research over ment of Health, Education, and Welfare have repeatedly referred to "the basic sciences related to processes of human growth and development." Although again these sciences are not specified, the series of reports makes the nature and scope of the NICHD program very clear: it is "focusing not on any one disease or part of the body but on the continuing process of growth and development, biological and behavioral, from reproduction and perinatal development, through infancy and childhood to maturation and aging." The same reports also set forth the broad range of social issues with which the Institute is concerned. These include the need to develop contraceptive methods that are, among other things, suited to the diverse requirements of the world's varied population groups; poor nutrition, and how it affects the childbearing woman and her progeny; the social, economic, and cultural factors that can contribute to mental retardation; the relationships between biological, social and environmental factors in aging; and such questions as how children acquire values and how changes in our culture affect personality structure.

As recently as April 1971, an editorial in the British journal *Developmental Medicine and Child Neurology,* in questioning certain current practices, suggested that they must displease "any true student of the developmental sciences," also without a further comment on this term. In view of the fact that important scientific and social issues have been made the province of the developmental sciences, the question, "What are the developmental sciences?" is certainly legitimate, indeed overdue.

Without trying to fathom the mystery of the sudden emergence of the developmental sciences or to probe into their past progress from mere observation to scientific conceptualization, methodology, research, theory, knowledge, and social application, this essay will suggest new bibliographic approaches to the literature currently evolving in this field. The processes of identifying this literature will be linked with an effort to find answers to the question of what the developmental sciences are. The analysis will be based on a sample drawn from the nearly one thousand bibliographic entries for books listed in the three latest volumes of the *Mental Health Book Review Index,* Volumes 14, 15, and 16, 1969-1971. These books were published during the period that coincides with the recognition of the developmental sciences as lying within the area of, and yet being or becoming separate from, the behavioral sciences–roughtly 1965 to 1970.

the past decade to an expanding awareness of the problems presented by a population with a long life expectancy.[71] Botwinick concludes his review of the research literature on *Cognitive Processes in Maturity and Old Age*[72] with a word of caution: ". . . through long life experience, older people may develop a degree of wisdom and sagacity not likely to be found in young people. The elements of wisdom and sagacity are not represented in the scientific data, and therefore, were not given the emphasis in this book they deserve." It will be important, therefore, to include in the developmental literature about the adult personality and the human life cycle works that represent the viewpoint of humanistic psychology and stress the processes of integration.[73-74]

The convergence of scientific and social concerns is again illustrated in two research reports, the first forming one of the Langley Porter Institute Studies of Aging, the second resulting from a proposal by the Committee on Older Persons of the Cleveland Welfare Federation.[75-76] Of the last three books on this subject in the present sample, one is limited to retirement, the others are more comprehensive, include theories of aging, and attempt to integrate diverse contributions.[77-79] One chapter in *Behavior and Adaptation in Late Life,* entitled "How the Old Face Death," illustrates the recent transition from gerontology to the study of death and dying.

Twenty books in the present sample deal wholly or in a significant part with death. Six of the books are concerned with suicide: the most comprehensive is *Suicidal Behaviors* with contributions by 48 authors, but even the slim monograph of the World Health Organization, *Prevention of Suicide,* shows that many countries share the rising concern about this problem.[80-81] Several other books deal with anxiety, bereavement, mourning, and other aspects of the problems surrounding death, as experienced by the living.[82-85,43] A book of unusually broad scope is *Man's Concern with Death,* by Toynbee and others.[86] Closest to the view that death is the final stage of the life cycle are Eissler's *The Psychiatrist and the Dying Patient,* first published in 1955, and recently reissued in a paperback edition, *Awareness of Dying* and *Time for Dying,* two studies resulting from a long-term research project, *Communication with the Fatally Ill,* and the account of an interdisciplinary academic program, *On Death and Dying* by Kübler-Ross.[87-91] A link between childhood and death is offered in a British study[92] and in *Psychological Emergencies of Childhood,* based in part on a study of children's reactions to the death of a parent and including a case report of a dying child in analysis at age four.[93]

## ISSUES AND CONCEPTS IN DEVELOPMENTAL THEORY AND RESEARCH

The growing interest in early determinants of development has drawn on and has further stimulated the study of animal behavior. The resulting books range in scope from a comprehensive review of research aimed at a synthesis of ethology and comparative psychology to a review of studies on *Imprinting and Early Learning.*[94–95] Increasingly, developmental animal research has been directed to exploring "the biodynamic roots of human behavior," but this is seldom as explicitly and succinctly suggested as in the proceedings of the American Academy of Psychoanalysis of 1967, entitled *Animal and Human.*[96–97] Indeed, the extent to which animal and human studies tend to be intertwined in books on early behavior and experience is usually not apparent from the titles which spell out the developmental orientation.[1–3,30,32,51] This is also true for books on more specific issues such as the origins and development of aggression, which has been approached from a variety of disciplines and perspectives, including neurology, psychiatry, ethology, psychology, and anthropology.[98–102]

The problem of applying findings from animal studies to human development is not easily resolved, however, and some attempts to do so have led to intense controversies. Nevertheless, the trend has been to draw together work on the study of developmental problems despite great diversity in origins and approaches. Harriet L. Rheingold, a coeditor of *Early Behavior; Comparative and Developmental Approaches,* sees in this work the possibility of a common area and a new division of knowledge: the development of behavior in immature organisms, man and animal, leading to "a unified science of development" (Ref. 30, p. 292).

The effects of mother-infant relations on development have also been extensively studied. *Attachment,* the first volume of Bowlby's two-volume work *Attachment and Loss,* is an outgrowth of research begun in the 1960's at the Tavistock Clinic and Tavistock Institute of Human Relations. The 24 reviews of this book cited in the present volume of the *Mental Health Book Review Index* show that it is of great current interest, with ramifications in many different fields.[103] In another first volume of a two-volume work, Mahler presents her concepts of human symbiosis and separation-individuation in their pathological aspects—infantile psychosis,[104] although she has also studied "the normal separation-individuation process." *Psychic Trauma* and *The Birth of the Ego* may further illustrate the developmental ramifications of contemporary psychoanalytic thinking.[105-106] The classical psychoanalytic theory of libido development is represented in the present sample through the coincidence of a recent reissue of papers first published five and six decades ago.[24] In discussing changing and current concepts, Escalona mentions Erikson's influence on the concept of developmental stages (Ref. 46, pp. 15-16). In a broad synthesis attempting to integrate concepts from three schools of thought—psychoanalysis, Heinz Werner, and Piaget—Arieti offers his own developmental viewpoint as an approach to "the intrapsychic self."[107]

Another concept that can potentially unify developmental studies conducted in diverse fields is "socialization," defined as the social process through which an individual becomes integrated into a social group. Although the term is sometimes limited to processes that occur in childhood, socialization, like development in the broader sense, has come to be seen as a life-long process. It is one of the concepts that may help to mark the fine line that separates the developmental from the behavioral sciences. Through a developmental approach, studies of attitude formation and change have turned into research on the socialization process and moral development, as conducted in England under the auspices of the Television Research Committee.[108] In this country, some large-scale attitude studies with school children have been concerned with political socialization.[23] Dawson and Prewitt state that "among the most significant questions about political socialization is: how does it fit into the individual life cycle," and they view "political socialization as a process that continues through the life span" (Ref. 109, pp. 41-42). The relevance of this work to current public issues such as the impact of television and the lowering of the voting age is obvious. A study of professional socialization in the field of nursing[110] is another example of the expanding scope and application of this concept.

Such related topics as social competence, societal expectations, and the social bases of adaptation and failures are treated in a book on human adaptation.[111] A British study using the Vineland Social Maturity Scale contains a chapter on the discrepancies between intelligence and social competence.[112] A much broader cross-cultural study with still another perspective has as its major objective "to explore the environmental and other factors which hinder the development of abilities within underdeveloped countries or depressed minority groups" (Ref. 113, p. 7).

A "developmental sequence" is illustrated by considering three books together: a comprehensive study of *The Development of Sex Differences, Sex and Gender,* which reports research on the development of masculinity and femininity, and *Transsexualism and Sex Reassignment,* which is concerned with a deviant development that can usually be traced to cross-gender identification in childhood.[20-21,114]

Sometimes the subjects used indicate the developmental orientation of the research, for example, twin studies.[115-116] A study of 106 preschool children, designed to predict reading failure, included 53 prematurely born children and thus provided data that throw light on problems of maturational lag.[117] Extensive case studies, for example, of the development of one child's personality or language,[44,118] may also provide valuable data and insights.

Child-rearing practices, child care, and child guidance have always been subjects in the borderland between the fields of child study and child development, depending on the emphasis of the research. In *The Children of the Dream,*[119] Bettelheim has added his observations to those made from time to time in earlier studies of Israeli children reared in a kibbutz. For various specific subjects, including foster care, adoption, and child abuse, the main effort is still directed toward ascertaining the basic facts. Perhaps most promising from the viewpoint of the developmental sciences are long-term and follow-up studies,[120-124] comprehensive reviews of research,[125] and multidisciplinary explorations.[126]

Research that contributes to an understanding of the influences of social and cultural conditions on human development also contributes to the social significance of the developmental sciences. It has had, and continues to have, an impact on national policy and important court decisions. A retrospective assessment of the social impact of the behavioral sciences may show that the research findings that have been translated into new national programs and legislation, such as school desegregation, the Headstart program, and the reform of adoption laws, grew out of work that would now be associated with the developmental sciences. Especially in the past two decades, growing scientific interest in human development has coincided with the growing awareness of the need to improve conditions and opportunities for the poor, the disadvantaged, and the deprived. Among the books that illustrate the merging of these trends are two reviews of the literature, *Low-Income Youth in Urban Areas* and *Growing Up Poor,*[127-128] *Children of Crisis,* an account of a psychiatrist's eight-year study based on interviews with Negro children in the South,[129] *The Drifters,* a long term study of children of disorganized lower-class families,[130] and two collections of papers, *The Disadvantaged Child* and *Social Class, Race, and Psychological Development.*[131,41] A new perspective was opened in 1967 by the international and multidisciplinary conference on *Malnutrition, Learning and Behavior,*[132] whose organizers, in the words of one reviewer, "directed attention to an urgent and persistent problem that confronts the world" (*Contemporary Psychology,* 1970, 15, 21).

## THE EVOLVING ORGANIZATION OF THE DEVELOPMENTAL SCIENCES

Finally, it would be timely to observe and study how the developmental sciences are organizing themselves. Although broad programs like those of NICHD and the Developmental Sciences Trust mentioned earlier provide a new focus for these processes, such organization requires a long preparation through small, often barely visible steps, for which the scientific community and concerned citizens and professionals take the initiative. One such sequence of steps, for example, takes the form of progressive recognition of the scientists and scholars who have made significant contributions to knowledge. In the field of developmental theory and research, a listing of those who have received lasting recognition would have to go back at least to Freud, G. Stanley Hall, and other late 19th-century pioneers in genetic psychology. Grinder's history of this field as "the first science of human development" includes

Darwin and even Aristotle.[12] The names of several contemporary authors of work that has been recognized as original, important, and influential appear in the present limited sample. To the books cited earlier (e.g., 5; 10; 27-29; 74; 99; 103) can be added further books by or about Piaget, Erikson, Sears, Anna Freud, and Kurt Lewin.[133-141]

A retrospective survey of the gradual organization of the developmental sciences is not within the scope of this essay. A few examples, however, will illustrate the trends that can currently be observed.

The present sample includes fourteen conferences, symposia, and society proceedings (Refs. 1-3; 11; 30; 33; 60; 61; 66; 97; 98; 102; 132; 147), and various volumes of invited papers (e.g., 27; 32; 79). Many of their organizers and contributors have worked at the frontiers of developmental research. That a new monographic series can focus on recently opened perspectives even in an older field is shown, for example, in the British series "Studies in Child Development," sponsored by the National Bureau for Co-operation in Child Care.[55,125,142-144] In the newly emerging field concerned with the scientific study of death, three journals were launched in 1970/71: *Omega,* published under the auspices of the Center for Psychological Studies of Dying, Death, and Lethal Behavior, Wayne State University; *Life-Threatening Behavior,* the official publication of the American Association of Suicidology; and the *Journal of Thanatology,* published by the Foundation of Thanatology, Columbia-Presbyterian Medical Center.

Institutions have played a vital role in the progress of the developmental sciences, by sponsoring conferences and publications and by providing the settings where the authors gained their pertinent experience or conducted their research. The programs of developmental studies of some institutions are already well-known, for example, those existing at the Tavistock and the Hampstead Child-Therapy Clinics in England, at the Menninger Foundation and the Langley Porter Neuropsychiatric Institute in this country (Refs. 103; 31; 140; 47; 75); others, such as the studies carried out at the Pediatric Language Disorder Clinic, Babies Hospital, Columbia-Presbyterian Medical Center, and at the Gender Identity Research Clinic at the University of California, Los Angeles, are made known through the authors' acknowledgments (Refs. 118; 21). An institution specifically dedicated to developmental studies may show this in its name, for example, the Laboratory of Human Development, Stanford University, the Child Development Center, New York City, and the Center for the Study of Aging and Human Development, Duke University (Refs. 139; 11; 79).

Organizations and special committees may recommend or initiate the conferences and literature surveys that bring new work on a subject into focus, for example, the Perinatal Research Committee established by the National Institute of Neurological Diseases and Blindness (Refs. 52; 30; 67). On a smaller scale, individual projects of limited duration can contribute to the emerging identity and organization of the developmental sciences.[58-59] Sometimes the names of such projects provide the main clue to the book's relevance to developmental research, for example, "Parental Influences on Early Ego Development in the Child" and "Child Rearing Practices Among Low Income Families in the District of Columbia."[145-146]

Innovations in the organization of science often begin outside of universities, but lead later to new centers and institutes in academic settings and ultimately to new disciplines or subdisciplines. Since the mid-1960's the transformation of older disciplines under the influence of the spreading developmental orientation has gathered momentum. So far, the trend has been not to strive from the start for a unified developmental science—an effort that was made for the behavioral sciences in the 1950's—but to recognize, within a field of specialization, a section that further specializes in a developmental approach. In recent years, there has been a marked increase in the use of the word "developmental" in a form suggesting a subdiscipline. An example was set earlier when the name of genetic psychology was changed to "developmental psychology." In titles of recent books and journals, anatomy, biology, cytology, genetics, immunology, medicine, neurobiology, neurology, and psychobiology are each preceded by the word "developmental."

One would be ill-advised, however, to define "the developmental sciences" according to such outward indicators. In addition to old disciplines such as embryology, various new disciplines that are also central to developmental research do not show this relevance in their names. Examples are behavior genetics[147] and teratology, which attained extraordinary social significance through the thalidomide crisis of the early 1960's and the intensified study of the causes of congenital malformations. Moreover, the bulk of work on developmental problems is still being done within the domain of one or another of the biomedical, psychological, and social sciences, without any organized differentiation.

In his Aldrich Award Address entitled "Child Development: a Basic Science for Pediatrics," presented in 1966 to the Section of Child Development of the American Academy of Pediatrics, Julius B. Richmond analyzed some of the issues that enter into the developmental reorientation of an established field. Pointing beyond the limits of his own specialty, he urged that "the concept of human development must become a central theme of medical education if it is to meet the changing needs of society." In light of the shift in the fields of human biology and medicine from an emphasis on disease to one on process, he proposed that "processes may be ordered around development as a unifying concept" (Ref. 9, pp. 141-142).

As has been shown earlier in this essay, the same thought underlies most efforts to come to grips with this new course of human affairs which has been equally and simultaneously spurred by three converging trends: scientific advances, the pressures of social needs and cultural crises, and the call on national governments and world bodies for programs designed to alleviate, if not to solve, the ensuing problems. Recognition of the developmental sciences, as here outlined, might help to reveal and to promote progress on each separate, as well as on the common, front.

## REFERENCES AND NOTES

1. Isaacson, Robert Lee, ed. *The neuropsychology of development; a symposium.* [Papers presented at the third of five special programs sponsored by the Department of Psychology of the University of Michigan in 1967 in honor of the University's 150th birthday. Contributors: Elliot S. Valenstein and others. Organizing Committee: N. R. F. Maier and others, Helen Peak, chairman. With reports and reviews of research and bibliographies.] N.Y., London, Wiley, 1968. 177 pp.

2. Ambrose, Anthony, ed. *Stimulation in early infancy; proceedings of a C.A.S.D.S. Study Group on "The Functions of Stimulation in Early Postnatal Development" held jointly with the Ciba Foundation, London, November 1967 . . .* N.Y., London, Academic Press, 1969. 289 pp. At head of title: Centre for Advanced Study in the Developmental Sciences.

3. Robinson, Roger James, ed. *Brain and early behaviour: development in the fetus and infant; proceedings of a C.A.S.D.S. Study Group on "Brain Mechanisms of Early Behavioural Development" held jointly with the Ciba Foundation, London, February 1968* . . . N.Y., London, Academic Press, 1969. 374 pp. At head of title: Centre for Advanced Study in the Developmental Sciences.

4. Harris, Dale B., ed. *The concept of development; an issue in the study of human behavior.* Minneapolis, Univ. of Minnesota Pr.; London, Oxford University Press, 1957. 287 pp.

5. Baldwin, Alfred Lee. *Theories of child development.* [Dedicated to the memory of Gordon S. Ierardi. With a bibliography.] N.Y., London, Wiley, 1966, © 1967. 618 pp.

6. Hoffman, Lois Norma Wladis, and Hoffman, Martin Leon, eds. *Review of child development research.* Vol. 2. [By Henry Borow and others.] Prepared under the auspices of the Society for Research in Child Development. [Advisory Committee: Nancy Bayley and others. Editorial consultants: Aline B. Auerbach and others. With bibliographies.] N.Y., Russell Sage Foundation, 1966. 598 pp. (Publications of Russell Sage Foundation.)

7. *Advances in child development and behavior.* Vol. 3, 1967. Edited by Lewis P. Lipsitt and Charles C. Spiker. Contributors: Robert J. Ellingson, Raymond H. Hohle, Herbert Kaye, Howard H. Kendler, Tracy S. Kendler, Robert E. Klein, Eleanor E. Maccoby, Anne D. Pick, Herbert L. Pick, Jr., and Michael D. Zeiler. [With bibliographies.] N.Y., London, Academic Press, 1967. 272 pp.

8. Brackbill, Yvonne, ed. *Infancy and early childhood; a handbook and guide to human development.* [Contributors: Alfred Steinschneider and others. With extensive reviews of the literature and bibliographies.] N.Y., Free Press; London, Collier-Macmillan, 1967. 523 pp.

9. *Annual progress in child psychiatry and child development.* [Vol. 1,] 1968. Edited by Stella Chess and Alexander Thomas. [Articles appearing in 1967. With an article by Peter H. Wolff, *The role of biological rhythms in early psychological development,* presented in an earlier version at the Menninger Foundation, October 1966, upon the occasion of the 1966 Helen Sargent memorial award. With an article by Julius B. Richmond, *Child development: a basic science for pediatrics,* presented on acceptance of the C. Anderson Aldrich award of 1966, Annual Meeting, Section on Child Development, American Academy of Pediatrics, October 23, 1966. With bibliographies.] N.Y., Brunner/Mazel, 1968, 565 pp.

10. Maier, Henry William. *Three theories of child development: the contributions of Erik H. Erikson, Jean Piaget, and Robert R. Sears, and*

*their applications.* Under the editorship of [and with an introd. by] Werner W. Boehm. [Foreword by Dale B. Harris. With bibliographies and an appendix: The complete works of the three theorists: Erik H. Erikson: 1930-1964; Jean Piaget: 1924-1964; Robert R. Sears: 1936-1961.] N.Y., London, Harper & Row, 1965. 314 pp.

11. Neubauer, Peter B., ed. *Concepts of development in early childhood education; an institute conducted by the Child Development Center, New York City* [in September, 1962. Four papers by David P. Ausubel, Lili E. Peller, Irving Sigel, and Jules Henry, with discussions by Millie Almy and others. With a bibliography.] Springfield, Ill., Thomas, 1965. 149 pp.

12. Grinder, Robert Eugene, ed. *A history of genetic psychology, the first science of human development.* [A collection of readings from ancient Greek to early 20th-century American sources, with commentary.] N.Y., London, Wiley, 1967. 247 pp.

13. Kuo, Jên-yüan. *The dynamics of behavior development; an epigenetic view,* by Zing-yang Kuo. [Based in part on the author's studies of the ontogeny of behavior in birds, dogs, and cats, carried out 1927-1936 and 1947-1965. With reviews of the literature and a bibliography.] N.Y., Random House, 1967. 240 pp. (Studies in psychology, PP34.)

14. Staats, Arthur Wilbur. *Learning, language, and cognition; theory, research, and method for the study of human behavior and its development.* [Based on the author's research conducted during the past twelve years. Dedicated to Pavlov and Thorndike. With a bibliography.] N.Y., London, Holt, Rinehart & Winston, 1968. 614 pp.

15. Lunzer, Eric Anthony. *Development in learning; behavior: learning: education.* [Vol.] 1: *The regulation of behaviour,* by E. A. Lunzer. [Contributors: E. A. Lunzer, N. Moray, and J. F. Morris. Dedicated to Jean Piaget. With reviews of the literature and bibliographies. [Vol.] 2: *Development in human learning.* Edited by E. A. Lunzer and J. F. Morris. [Contributors: M. Blank, P. Herriot, H. Kay, M. M. Lewis, K. Lovell, E. A. Lunzer, J. F. Morris, E. A. Peel, G. F. Reed, G. R. Roberts, H. R. Schaeffer, R. R. Skemp, and M. D. Vernon. With reviews of the literature and bibliographies. [Vol.] 3: *Contexts of education.* Edited by J. F. Morris and E. A. Lunzer. [Contributors: W. A. L. Blyth, H. J. Butcher, A. Cashdan, A. D. B. Clarke, D. H. Hargreaves, E. A. Lunzer, J. F. Morris, D. H. Stott, and F. W. Warburton. With reviews of the literature and bibliographies.] N.Y., American Elsevier; London, Staples Press, 1968-1969. 3v.

16. Fellows, Brian John. *The discrimination process and development.* [With reviews of the literature and a bibliography.] N.Y., Oxford, Pergamon Press, 1968. 218 pp. (International series of mono-

graphs in experimental psychology, vol. 5)

17. Kidd, Aline Halstead, and Rivoire, Jeanne L., eds. *Perceptual development in children.* [Contributors: Louise B. Ames and others. Pref. by Edna Heidbreder. Introd. by Gardner Murphy. With reviews of the literature and of research in progress and with bibliographies.] N.Y., International Universities Press, 1966; London, Univ. of London Pr., 1967. 548 pp.

18. Warren, Richard M., and Warren, Roslyn P. *Helmholtz on perception: its physiology and development.* [Selections, with prefatory comments. With a sketch of Helmholtz's life and work and a bibliography.] N.Y., London, Wiley, 1968. 277 pp.

19. Völgyesi, Ferenc András. *Hypnosis of man and animals, with special reference to the development of the brain in the species and the individual.* 2d ed., rev. in collaboration with the author by Gerhard Klumbies. [Translated from the German, Menschen- und Tierhypnose, 2d ed., Zürich, 1963, by M. W. Hamilton. Introd. to the English ed. by A. Spencer Paterson. With a survey of the history of animal hypnosis, reviews of the literature, and a bibliography.] London, Baillière, Tindall & Cassell, 1966; Baltimore, Williams & Wilkins, © 1966. 216 pp.

20. Maccoby, Eleanor Emmons, ed. *The development of sex differences.* [Outgrowth of the discussions of a work group that met at Stanford University, 1962-1964, sponsored by the Committee on Socialization and Social Structure of the Social Science Research Council.] With contributions by Roy G. D'Andrade, Sanford M. Dornbusch, David A. Hamburg, Lawrence Kohlberg, Donald T. Lunde, Eleanor E. Maccoby, Walter Mischel, and Roberta M. Oetzel. With a classified summary of research in sex differences. With an annotated bibliography compiled by Roberta M. Oetzel. With reviews of the literature and bibliographies.] Stanford, Calif., Stanford Univ. Pr., 1966; London, Tavistock, 1967. 351 pp. (Stanford studies in psychology, 5.)

21. Stoller, Robert Jesse. *Sex and gender; on the development of masculinity and femininity.* [A clinical report of the author's research conducted over ten years in the Gender Identity Research Clinic at the University of California, Los Angeles, with the collaboration of Howard J. Baker and others. Based on a study of 85 patients, primarily white, middle-class Americans, and 63 members of their families. With extensive case reports and an appendix: Data on transsexuals. With a bibliography.] N.Y., Science House, 1968. 383 pp. London, Hogarth Press & Institute of Psycho-Analysis, 1968. 383 pp. (The International psycho-analytical library, no. 81.)

22. Flavell, John Hurley. *The development of role-taking and communication skills in children.* In collaboration with Patricia T. Botkin,

Charles L. Fry, Jr., John W. Wright and Paul E. Jarvis. [A report of the authors' studies conducted with various groups of school children in middle childhood and adolescence and with samples of children at ages one to seven. With a survey of previous theory and research and a bibliography.] N.Y., London, Wiley, 1968. 239 pp.

23. Hess, Robert Daniel, and Torney, Judith V. *The development of political attitudes in children.* [Report of a study begun at the University of Chicago in 1960, John David Jackson, project director, conducted in eight cities in four different regions of the United States. Based on interviews of 5,000 children and on questionnaires given to 12,000 elementary school children in grades 2 to 8. Outgrowth of a number of studies of political socialization conducted by Robert D. Hess and David Eaton. With excerpts from the tape-recorded interviews and a bibliography.] Chicago, London, Aldine, 1967. 288 pp. Paperback ed.: Garden City, N.Y., Anchor Books, Doubleday, 1968. 331 pp. (A Doubleday anchor book, A640.)

24. Abraham, Karl. *On character and libido development; six essays* [originally published 1911-1925, reprinted from the author's Selected papers, London, 1927, N.Y., 1953]. Edited with an introd. by Bertram D. Lewin. Translated [from the German] by Douglas Bryan and Alix Strachey. [With a bibliography.] N.Y., Basic Books, 1966. 206 pp. Paperback ed.: N.Y., Norton, 1966. 206 pp. (The Norton library, N316.)

25. Stephenson, Geoffrey M. *The development of conscience.* [Based on the author's thesis, University of Nottingham, with title: Conscience and psychopathy. With examples from the author's studies of twenty psychopaths, aged seventeen to twenty-five, and 100 non-psychopathic fifteen-year old boys. With a bibliography.] N.Y., Humanities Press; London, Routledge & Paul, 1966. 134 pp. (International library of sociology and social reconstruction.)

26. Kay, William. *Moral development; a psychological study of moral growth from childhood to adolescence.* [Based largely on a survey and analysis of the research literature, 1925-1960.] With a foreword by John Wilson. [With bibliographies.] London, Allen & Unwin, 1968; N.Y., Schocken Books, 1969. 270 pp. Paperback ed.: London, Allen & Unwin, 1968. 270 pp. (Unwin university books.)

27. Elkind, David, and Flavell, John Hurley, eds. *Studies in cognitive development; essays in honor of Jean Piaget.* [Contributors: Harry Beilin and others. With reviews of the literature and bibliographies.] N.Y., London, Oxford Univ. Pr., 1969. 503 pp.

28. Piaget, Jean. *On the development of memory and identity.* [Two lectures, "Memory and operations of intelligence," based on a book then in press with title Mémoire et intelligence by J. Piaget and

B. Inhelder in collaboration with H. Sinclair, Paris, 1968, and "Identity and conservation," based on a volume of Études d'épistémologie génétique, Paris, 1968.] Translated by Eleanor Duckworth. [With a pref.: The Heinz Werner lecture series, by Bernard Kaplan, Seymour Wapner, and Joachim F. Wohlwill. The second volume in the lecture series, sponsored by the Heinz Werner Institute of Developmental Psychology, Clark University. With a bibliography.] Worcester, Mass., Clark Univ. Pr. with Barre Publishers, 1968. 42 pp. (Heinz Werner lectures, 1967.)

29. Beard, Ruth Mary. *An outline of Piaget's developmental psychology for students and teachers.* [Series editor's foreword by Ben Morris. With extensive examples of Piaget's observations and a bibliography.] N.Y., Basic Books, 1969. 139 pp. London, Routledge & Paul, 1969. 128 pp. (The Student's library of education.)

30. Stevenson, Harold William, Hess, Eckard Heinrich, and Rheingold, Harriet Lange, eds. *Early behavior: comparative and developmental approaches.* [Essays based on two research conferences held in 1963 and 1965 by the Committee on Comparative-Developmental Behavior, Harold W. Stevenson, chairman, organized in 1961 by the Social Science Research Council. Contributors: Erich Klinghammer, Byron A. Campbell, J. M. Warren, William A. Mason, Irenäus Eibl-Eibesfeldt, William Kessen, Robert L. Franz, Lewis P. Lipsitt, and Hanus Papoušek. With reviews of the literature and bibliographies.] N.Y., London, Wiley, 1967. 303 pp.

31. Nagera, Humberto. *Early childhood disturbances, the infantile neurosis, and the adulthood disturbances; problems of a developmental psychoanalytic psychology.* [Part of a study entitled "Assessment of Pathology in Childhood," conducted at the Hampstead Child Therapy Clinic and Course, London. Dedicated to Anna Freud. Foreword by Anna Freud. With case examples and a bibliography.] N.Y., International Universities Press, 1966; London, Hogarth Press, 1967. 95 pp. (The Psychoanalytic Study of the Child. Monograph no. 2.)

32. Newton, Grant, and Levine, Seymour, eds. *Early experience and behavior; the psychobiology of development.* [Contributors: Ilya A. Arshavsky and others. With reviews of the research literature and bibliographies.] Springfield, Ill., Thomas, 1968. 785 pp.

33. Zubin, Joseph, and Jervis, George Amedee, eds. *Psychopathology of mental development; the proceedings of the Fifty-sixth Annual Meeting of the American Psychopathological Association, held in New York City, February 1966.* [With an introductory sketch: George A. Jervis, Samuel W. Hamilton memorial lecturer, 1966, by Elaine F. Kinder. With the Samuel W. Hamilton memorial award lecture for 1966: Some observations on the problem of heredity and environment in men-

tal retardation, by George A. Jervis. With the presidential address by Seymour S. Kety: Intelligence, biology and social responsibility. With reviews of the literature and bibliographies.] N.Y., Grune & Stratton; London, Heinemann Medical Books [distributor], 1967. 658 pp.

34. Wood, Nancy Elizabeth. *Delayed speech and language development.* [Series editor's note by Charles Van Riper. With a bibliography.] Englewood Cliffs, N.J., London, Prentice-Hall, 1964. 142 pp. (Foundations of speech pathology series.)

35. Rawson, Margaret B. *Developmental language disability; adult accomplishments of dyslexic boys.* [Report of a study of the 56 boys, dyslexics and nondyslexics, between six and fourteen years of age, representing 44 families, who attended The School in Rose Valley, Moylan, Pennsylvania, for at least three of their elementary years during the period between 1930 and 1947, and of a follow-up study based on 86 interviews with the subjects or other informants, conducted 1964-1965 when the boys' ages ranged from twenty-six to forty years. Based on the author's professional experience with dyslexic children since 1935. With case reports, a brief survey of the literature, and a selected bibliography.] Baltimore, Johns Hopkins Press; London, Oxford Univ. Pr. [distributor], 1968. 127 pp. (Hood College monograph series, no. 2.)

36. Cowie, Valerie Aileen. *A study of the early development of mongols.* [An abridged form of a Ph.D thesis, University of London, 1967. Based largely on a study of the early infantile reflexes in the first ten months of life of 79 babies with mongolism born over thirteen months, 1963-1964. Introd. by Brian H. Kirman. Pref. by R. G. Mitchell. With reviews of the literature and a bibliography.] N.Y., Oxford, Published for the Institute for Research into Mental Retardation by Pergamon Press, 1970. 110 pp. (Institute for Research into Mental Retardation. Monograph, no. 1.)

37. Llorens, Lela A., and Rubin, Eli Zunder. *Developing ego functions in disturbed children: occupational therapy in milieu.* [Outgrowth of six years of experimental work at Lafayette Clinic, Detroit, in the development of programs in occupational therapy for disturbed children in residential treatment. With bibliographies.] Detroit, Wayne State University, 1967. 146 pp. (Lafayette Clinic handbooks in psychiatry, no. 1.)

38. D'Amato, Gabriel. *Residential treatment for child mental health; towards ego-social development and a community-child model.* [Based in part on the author's experience as child psychiatrist at Eastern State School and Hospital, Trevose, Pennsylvania, opened in 1962.] With a foreword by Joseph Adlestein. [With case material, reviews of

the literature, and a bibliography.] Springfield, Ill., Thomas, 1969. 186 pp.

39. Senn, Milton John Edward, and Solnit, Albert J. *Problems in child behavior and development.* [Based on the authors' work with parents and children in distress at the Yale Child Study Center. With case material and a bibliography.] Philadelphia, Lea & Febiger: London, Kimpton, 1968. 268 pp.

40. Ratcliffe, Thom Arundel. *The development of personality.* [Outgrowth of the author's advisory collaboration with the "in-service" training program at the National Marriage Guidance Council and of his experience during the past fifteen years in conducting lecture courses at universities and training programs for nurses, health visitors, teachers, and social case-workers.] N.Y., Humanities Press; London, Allen & Unwin, 1967. 118 pp.

41. Deutsch, Martin, Katz, Irwin, and Jensen, Arthur Robert, eds. *Social class, race, and psychological development.* [Papers by I. I. Gottesman and others, with introductions by the editors. Dedicated to the memory of Dr. Martin Luther King, Jr. Pref. by Ernest R. Hilgard. Sponsored by the Society for the Psychological Study of Social Issues. With reviews of the literature and bibliographies.] N.Y., London, Holt, Rinehart & Winston, 1968. 423 pp.

42. Blanck, Rubin, and Blanck, Gertrude. *Marriage and personal development.* [Based in part on the senior author's experience with marital counseling over a period of many years. With case illustrations and a bibliography.] N.Y., London, Columbia Univ. Pr., 1968, 191 pp.

43. Moriarty, David Michael. *The loss of loved ones; the effects of a death in the family on personality development,* compiled and edited by David M. Moriarty. With contributions, [papers and discussions written in response to Part I, the author's manuscript] by Timothy Harrington, Albert Krinsky, Bernard Rosenblatt, Sebastiano Santostefano, John Scott, Elvin Semrad, Gordon Torgerson, and Carl Wahlstrom. With a foreword by Bardwell H. Flower. [With extensive case material and transcripts of interviews with psychiatric patients at Worcester State Hospital. With bibliographies.] Springfield, Ill., Thomas, 1967. 203 pp.

44. Axline, Virginia Mae. *Dibs: in search of self; personality development in play therapy.* [A complete case history of the psychological development of one boy. Under the editorship of, and with an introd. by, Leonard Carmichael.] Boston, Houghton Mifflin, 1964; London, Gollancz, 1966. 186 pp. Paperback ed.: With an introd. by Leonard Carmichael. N.Y., Ballantine Books, 1967. 220 pp.

45. Bijou, Sidney William, and Baer, Donald Merle. *Child development.* Vol. 2: *Universal stage of infancy.* [With reviews of the literature and bibliographies.] N.Y., Appleton-Century-Crofts, 1965. 183 pp. (The Century psychology series.)

46. Escalona, Sibylle Korsch. *The roots of individuality; normal patterns of development in infancy.* [Outgrowth of the author's research conducted from 1944 to the mid-1960's. Based on the intensive analysis of 32 infant subjects, four to thirty-two weeks old, selected from 128 normal infants studied in an earlier research project published by the author and others as *Early phases of personality development,* Evanston, Ill., 1953. Dedicated to Kurt Lewin, David Rapaport, and John Benjamin. With case studies, a review of the research literature and a bibliography.] Chicago, Aldine, 1968. 547 pp. (Modern applications in psychology.) London, Tavistock, 1968. 547 pp.

47. Gardner, Riley Wetherell, and Moriarty, Alice Ewell. *Personality development at preadolescence; explorations of structure formation.* [Report of a study of 29 boys and 31 girls, aged nine to thirteen, from the Topeka, Kansas, area, drawn from a larger group of children studied in infancy by Sibylle Escalona and others. Outgrowth of the collaboration of two research groups at the Menninger Foundation, the Cognition Project, directed by the first author, and the Longitudinal Study Project, directed by the second author. Based on the use of various tests and measurements, including the Holtzman Inkblot Test, the Wechsler Intelligence Scale for Children, and ratings of overall behavior in the test situations. With case studies of two boys and two girls, one each high, the other low in ego strength. With reviews of the literature and a bibliography.] Seattle, Univ. of Washington Pr., 1968. 344 pp.

48. Lidz, Theodore. *The person: his development throughout the life cycle.* [With case illustrations and bibliographies.] N.Y., Basic Books; London, Harper & Row [distributor], 1968. 574 pp.

49. Biddle, William Wishart. *The community development process; the rediscovery of local initiative.* With the collaboration of Loureide J. Biddle. [Based in part on the authors' experience as community developers. With case studies of development projects in two communities, a mining county in rural Appalachia and a deteriorating neighborhood in a northern industrial city, 1957-1960. With an appendix: Community development in the United States and in Canada and Puerto Rico. With bibliographies.] N.Y., London, Holt, Rinehart & Winston, 1965. 334 pp.

50. Pye, Lucian Wilmot. *The spirit of Chinese politics; a psycho-*

*cultural study of the authority crisis in political development.* [An essay using information obtained by the author in a study, published as his Guerrilla communism in Malaya, Princeton, N.J., 1956, and in a study of Chinese communism carried out in Hong Kong in 1964. Dedicated to Max F. Millikan.] Cambridge, Mass., London, M.I.T. Press, 1968. 255 pp.

51. Joffe, J. M. *Prenatal determinants of behaviour.* [Outgrowth and expansion of a review of work on prenatal influences included in the author's Ph.D. thesis. Series editor's introd. by H. J. Eysenck. With a report of the author's research carried out in the Institute of Psychiatry Animal Psychology Laboratory at the Bethlem Royal Hospital. With a bibliography.] N.Y., Oxford, Pergamon Press, 1969. 366 pp. (International series of monographs in experimental psychology. vol. 7.)

52. Richardson, Stephen Alexander, and Guttmacher, Alan Frank, eds. *Childbearing: its social and psychological aspects.* [A series of critical reviews, by Elaine R. Grimm, Ernest M. Gruenberg, Raymond Illsley, Margaret Mead, Niles Newton, and Jay S. Rosenblatt, of studies of reproduction oriented toward a social-science viewpoint. Outgrowth of a recommendation of the Perinatal Research Committee, established by the National Institute of Neurological Diseases and Blindness. Published under the auspices of the Association for the Aid of Crippled Children. With bibliographies.] Baltimore, Williams & Wilkins; Edinburgh, Livingstone [distributor], 1967. 334 pp.

53. Ainsworth, Mary Dinsmore Salter. *Infancy in Uganda; infant care and the growth of love.* [A report of research into the development of a sample of 28 Ganda infants, age two to fifteen months, undertaken during the author's association with the East African Institute of Social Research in Kampala, Uganda, 1954-1955. Based on repeated visits with the families. Foreword by John Bowlby. With case summaries of the infants and their families. With a bibliography.] Baltimore, Johns Hopkins Press; London, Oxford Univ. Pr. [distributor], 1967. 471 pp.

54. Brackbill, Yvonne, and Thompson, George Greene, eds. *Behavior in infancy and early childhood; a book of readings* [1907-1966, with commentary. With case studies, reviews of the literature, and bibliographies.] N.Y., Free Press; London, Collier-Macmillan, 1967. 692 pp.

55. Pringle, Mia Lilly Kellmer, Butler, Neville R., and Davie, R. *11,000 seven-year olds;* first report of the National Child Development Study (1958 Cohort), submitted to the Central Advisory Council for Education (England), April 1966. Sponsored by the Institute of Child

Health, University of London, National Birthday Trust Fund, National Bureau for Co-operation in Child Care, National Foundation for Educational Research in England and Wales, in collaboration with the Association of Chief Education Officers (in England and Wales), Society of Medical Officers of Health, Association of Directors of Education (in Scotland). [Interim report produced after nineteen months in a three-year project, begun in October 1964, potentially the second stage of a longitudinal study of 17,000 babies born during the week, 3rd to 9th March 1958 in England, Scotland, and Wales. Based on information received for children in England by the middle of August 1965, from schools, mothers, and school health services, including educational data for 10,833 of these children and 7,985 completed Parental and Medical Questionnaires. Foreword by W. D. Wall, chairman of the Steering Committee. Consultative Committee: Sir Lionel Russell, chairman. With bibliographies.] London, Longmans, 1966; N.Y., Humanities Press, 1967. 246 pp. (Studies in child development.)

56. Thomas, Alexander, Chess, Stella, and Birch, Herbert George. *Temperament and behavior disorders in children.* [Report of a study of a clinical sample of 42 children with behavioral disturbances in the authors' longitudinal study of 136 children begun in 1956. With case histories and a selective extraction of data from the longitudinal records. With bibliographies.] N.Y., New York Univ. Pr.; London, Univ. of London Pr., 1968. 309 pp.

57. Masterson, James Francis, Jr. *The psychiatric dilemma of adolescence.* [Report of the Symptomatic Adolescent Research Project, a five-year study of 72 adolescent outpatients, average age on first examination 16, conducted 1956-1962 at Cornell University Medical College and the Payne Whitney Psychiatric Clinic, New York Hospital. With extensive case illustrations and a bibliography.] Boston, Little, Brown; London, Churchill, 1967. 217 pp.

58. Offer, Daniel. *The psychological world of the teen-ager; a study of normal adolescent boys.* [Report of the Modal Adolescent Project begun in 1961 and conducted over the four years of high school with 73 students in two suburban high schools in Chicago. Based on the Self-Image Questionnaire constructed at the National Opinion Research Center of the University of Chicago, and on interviews and psychological testing administered 1963-1966.] With the collaboration of Melvin Sabshin, and the assistance of Judith L. Offer. [With case illustrations and a bibliography.] N.Y., Basic Books; London, Harper & Row [distributor], 1969. 286 pp.

59. Group for the Advancement of Psychiatry. Committee on

Adolescence. *Normal adolescence: its dynamics and impact.* Formulated by the Committee on Adolescence, [Calvin F. Settlage, chairman. Dedicated to the memory of Joseph J. Michaels. With an appendix: Endocrinology of adolescence; sequence of pubertal phenomena; development of secondary sex characteristics. With a bibliography.] N.Y., Group for the Advancement of Psychiatry, 1968. pp. 745-858. (Group for the Advancement of Psychiatry. Report no. 68; Reports and symposiums, vol. 6, no. 9.) Another ed.: N.Y., Scribner, 1968. 127 pp.

60. Caplan, Gerald, and Lebovici, Serge, eds. *Adolescence: psychosocial perspectives.* [Based on clinical information and research results derived from current studies of adolescents in the United States and Europe, described and discussed by leading clinicians and researchers from eleven countries at the Sixth International Congress of Child Psychiatry, Edinburgh, July 1966. The authors: W. H. Allchin and others. Dedicated to the memory of Frederick H. Allen. A successor to *Emotional problems of early childhood,* edited by Gerald Caplan, N.Y., 1955, and *Prevention of mental disorders in children: initial explorations,* edited by Gerald Caplan, N.Y., 1961. With case material and bibliographies.] N.Y., Basic Books; London, Harper & Row [distributor], 1969. 412 pp.

61. Society for the Study of Addiction to Alcohol and Other Drugs. *The pharmacological and epidemiological aspects of adolescent drug dependence; proceedings* [of the first International Symposium] of the Society for the Study of Addiction, London, 1 and 2 September 1966. [Contributors: Simon Albury and others.] Edited by C. W. M. Wilson. [With a summary of the symposium by Roy Goulding. With summaries of the regulations controlling dangerous drugs in certain countries. With a glossary of slang terms used by addicts in the United Kingdom, reviews of the literature, and bibliographies.] N.Y., Oxford, Symposium Publications Division, Pergamon Press, 1968. 515 pp.

62. Schofield, Michael George. *The sexual behaviour of young people.* [Report of the author's research, begun in 1960, carried out under the auspices of the Central Council for Health Education, J. D. Kershaw, chairman of the Steering Committee. Based on interviews with 934 single boys and 939 single girls, aged fifteen to nineteen, in London and other English cities.] In collaboration with John Bynner, Patricia Lewis, and Peter Massie. [Foreword by Sir Herbert Broadley. With data on research into sex behavior, 1915-1964. With a bibliography.] Boston, Little, Brown; London, Longmans, Green, 1965. 316 pp.

63. *Minority group adolescents in the United States.* [Contributors:]

Eugene B. Brody, Robert L. Derbyshire, Stanley, L. M. Fong, Daniel Freeman, Chester M. Pierce, Edward Preble, Walter Weintraub, and Joe Yamamoto. [An introductory essay by Eugene B. Brody: *Adolescents as a United States minority group in an era of social change*, and a series of research based papers, mainly concerning Negro, Mexican, Puerto Rican, Oriental, and American Indian adolescents. With case material and bibliographies.] Baltimore, Williams & Wilkins, 1968. 243 pp.

64. Wittenberg, Rudolph M. *Postadolescence; theoretical and clinical aspects of psychoanalytic therapy.* [A volume in a series under the consultant editorship of Leopold Bellak. With case illustrations and a bibliography.] N.Y., Grune & Stratton; London, Heinemann Medical Books [distributor], 1968. 138 pp.

65. Wittenberg, Rudolph M. *The troubled generation; toward understanding and helping the young adult.* [Based on the author's experience over twenty-five years in psychoanalytic practice and as consultant to social agencies and clinics. With fictionalized case reports of six young people.] N.Y., Association Press, 1967. 192 pp.

66. Sherif, Muzafer, and Sherif, Carolyn Wood, eds. *Problems of youth: transition to adulthood in a changing world.* [Based on papers delivered by David P. Ausubel and others May 1964, at the Fifth Social Psychology Symposium held at the University of Oklahoma and organized by the Institute of Group Relations. With case examples, reviews of the literature, and bibliographies.] Chicago, Aldine, 1965. 336 pp. (Modern applications in psychology.)

67. Soddy, Kenneth, and Kidson, Mary C., eds. *Men in middle life.* Based on the study made by the one-time Scientific Committee of the World Federation for Mental Health. [A discussion of data derived from a survey of the literature relevant to the forty to sixty age period. Dedicated to the memory of Henricus Cornelius Rümke. Pref. by H. C. Rümke. With a bibliography of works in the English language, compiled by Frances Murphy and Sister Mary Cabrini Delahunty, and a bibliography of works in other languages, compiled by Ida Cermak.] Philadelphia, Lippincott [distributor]; London, Tavistock, 1967. 485 pp. (Cross-cultural studies in mental health, 3.)

68. Neugarten, Bernice Levin, ed. *Middle age and aging; a reader in social psychology.* [Papers reprinted, abridged, or adapted from previous publications, 1956-1968, and four previously unpublished papers, with commentary. Contributors: C. Knight Aldrich and others. Dedicated to the memory of Raymond G. Kuhlen. With reports and reviews of research and an extensive bibliography.] Chicago, London, Univ. of Chicago Pr., 1968. 596 pp.

69. Heron, Alastair, and Chown, Sheila M. *Age and function.* [Report of a study, conducted 1959-1963, of 50 men and 40 women in the age range from twenty to seventy-nine, forming the M.R.C. Merseyside Voluntary Research Panel.] Assisted by Staff of the Medical Research Council Unit for Research on Occupational Aspects of Ageing, Liverpool. With a foreword by G. E. W. Wolstenholme. [With an appendix: Smoking and age. With reviews of the literature and a bibliography.] Boston, Little, Brown; London, Churchill, 1967. 182 pp.

70. Bromley, Dennis Basil. *The psychology of human ageing.* [Editorial foreword by B. M. Foss. With an appendix: Methodological problems. With a bibliography.] Baltimore; Harmondsworth, Middlesex, Penguin Books, 1966. 365 pp. (Pelican books, A848; a Pelican original.)

71. Talland, George Alexander, ed. *Human aging and behavior; recent advances in research and theory.* [Contributors: Robert E. Canestrari, Jr., F. I. M. Craik, D. R. Davies, Carl Eisdorfer, Patrick Rabbitt, Klaus F. Riegel, K. Warner Schaie, Charles R. Strother, Walter W. Surwillo, Jacek Szafran, and George A. Talland. With bibliographies.] N.Y., London, Academic Press, 1968. 322 pp.

72. Botwinick, Jack. *Cognitive processes in maturity and old age.* [With reviews of the literature and bibliographies.] N.Y., Springer, 1967. 212 pp.

73. Arasteh, A. Reza. *Final integration in the adult personality; a measure for health, social change, and leadership.* [Completed after the response to the author's presentation of a brief report at the 17th International Congress of Psychology, Washington, D.C., August 1963, published with title: *Final integration in the adult personality,* Washington, 1963. With a psycho-cultural analysis of Rumi and of Goethe and a critique of Kurt R. Eissler's Goethe; a psychoanalytic study, Detroit, 1963. With reviews of the related literature and bibliographies.] N.Y., Heinman; Leiden, Brill, 1965. 404 pp.

75. Bühler, Charlotte Malachowski, and Massarik, Fred, eds. *The course of human life; a study of goals in the humanistic perspective.* Authors: James F. T. Bugental, Charlotte Bühler [and others. With case illustrations, reviews of the literature, and bibliographies.] N.Y., Springer, 1968. 422 pp.

75. Lowenthal, Marjorie Fiske, Berkman, Paul L., and associates. *Aging and mental disorder in San Francisco; a social psychiatric study.* [Report of one of a series of studies on aging conducted at the Langley Porter Neuropsychiatric Institute, California Department of Mental Hygiene and the Department of Psychiatry, University of California

School of Medicine, San Francisco, begun in 1958. Based on a study of 534 elderly first admissions to the psychiatric wards of the San Francisco General Hospital and on field work with a 600-case community sample of persons, sixty and older, in San Francisco, carried out by the Survey Research Center of the University of California, Berkeley.] By Marjorie Fiske Lowenthal and Paul L. Berkman and associates Gerard G. Brissette, John A. Buehler, Robert C. Pierce, Betsy C. Robinson, and Mella L. Trier. [With case illustrations, a bibliography, and a list of selected Project publications.] San Francisco, Jossey-Bass, 1967. 341 pp. (The Langley Porter Institute studies of aging.)

76. Rosow, Irwing. *Social integration of the aged.* [Report of research proposed by the Committee on Older Persons of the Cleveland Welfare Federation and conducted under joint auspices of Western Reserve University and the Federation. Based on an interview study of 1,200 middle-class and working-class men and women, mostly sixty-five years or older, residents of several hundred Cleveland apartment buildings. With an appendix: Housing dissatisfaction. With a review of the literature and a bibliography.] N.Y., Free Press; London, Collier-Macmillan, 1967. 354 pp.

77. Geist, Harold. *The psychological aspects of retirement.* With a foreword by Del E. Webb. [With reviews of pertinent studies and a bibliography.] Springfield, Ill., Thomas, 1968. 131 pp.

78. Burch, Philip Robert James. *An inquiry concerning growth, disease and ageing.* [Based on the author's unified theory of the pertinent physiological and pathological phenomena. With a historical survey of the unified theory, reviews of the research literature, and a bibliography.] Edinburgh, Oliver & Boyd, 1968; Toronto, Univ. of Toronto Pr., 1969. 213 pp.

79. Busse, Ewald William, and Pfeiffer, Eric, eds. *Behavior and adaptation in late life,* by 17 authors, [Kurt W. Back and others. Based in part on two longitudinal studies carried out at Duke University, the first initiated in 1954, entitled "The Effect of Aging upon the Central Nervous System," the second recently initiated, entitled "Adaptation to Change." With reviews of the literature and bibliographies.] Boston, Little, Brown; London, Churchill, 1969. 395 pp.

80. Resnik, Harvey Louis Paul. *Suicidal behaviors; diagnosis and management,* by 48 authors, [William F. Anderson and others. Foreword by Kenneth E. Appel.] Edited [and with a chapter: A community anti-suicide organization: the Friends of Dade County, Florida] by H. L. P. Resnik. [With case material, reviews of the literature, and a bibliography.] Boston, Little, Brown; London, Churchill, 1968. 536 pp.

81. World Health Organization. *Prevention of suicide.* [Outgrowth of discussions of suicide prevention in various countries, begun in 1966. Participants: T. Asuni, N. L. Farberow, P. Kielholz, E. Ringel, P. Sainsbury, E. Stengel, and P. M. Yap. A synthesis of an expanded report by N. L. Farberow and P. Sainsbury, with a review of the literature by the WHO Secretariat. With a bibliography.] Geneva, World Health Organization; London, H.M.S.O., 1968. 84 pp. (*Its* Public Health papers, no. 35.)

82. Rheingold, Joseph Cyrus. *The mother, anxiety, and death; the catastrophic death complex.* [With reviews of the literature and a bibliography.] Boston, Little, Brown; London, Churchill, 1967. 271 pp.

83. Gorer, Geoffrey. *Death, grief, and mourning in contemporary Britain.* [Based on survey interviews with a sample of 359 men and women over sixteen, carried out by Research Services Ltd., and on 80 longer reinterviews conducted by the author with the assistance of David Tomlinson, 1963. With extensive excerpts from interviews. With an autobiographical introd. With appendixes: Current and recent theories of mourning and the present material. Religious beliefs and practices: 1963 and 1950 compared. The pornography of death, first published in *Encounter,* October 1955. With a bibliography.] London, Cresset Press, 1965. 184 pp. American paperback ed. with title: *Death, grief, and mourning.* [With an introd. to the American ed.] Garden City, N.Y., Anchor Books, Doubleday, 1967. 205 pp. (A Doubleday anchor book, A555.)

84. Kutscher, Austin H., ed. *Death and bereavement,* edited by Austin H. Kutscher in collaboration with 49 contributors [Gene E. Bartlett and others] and 122 consultant-respondents [Richard B. Adams and others. Companion volume to the author's *But not to lose,* N.Y., 1969. With a selected anthology of the classical literature, by Sandra Bess. With a bibliography: Grief and bereavement: a selected annotated bibliography of behavioral science and psychiatric writings, by Richard A. Kalish. With case illustrations and bibliographies.] Springfield, Ill., Thomas, 1969. 364 pp.

85. Sudnow, David. *Passing on.* [Report of a study of "death work" undertaken 1963-1965 as a doctoral dissertation at the University of California, Berkeley, under the direction of Erving Goffman. Based on the author's field observations in County Hospital, *pseud.,* a large, urban West Coast charity institution, and Cohen Hospital, *pseud.,* a Midwestern, private, general hospital. With a survey of the literature and a bibliography.] Englewood Cliffs, N.J., Prentice-Hall, 1967. 212 pp. Paperback ed. with subtitle: *The social organization of dying.* [A more extended and analytic presentation of the findings

written for the sociologist.] Englewood Cliffs, N.J., London, Prentice-Hall, 1967. 176 pp.

86. *Man's concern with death* [by] Arnold Toynbee, A. Keith Mant, Ninian Smart, John Hinton, Simon Yudkin, Eric Rhode, Rosalind Heywood, and H. H. Price. [Publisher's foreword by Robin Denniston. With surveys of definitions and concepts of, and attitudes toward, death and with a chapter: Death in twentieth-century fiction, by Eric Rhode.] London, Hodder & Stoughton, 1968; N.Y., McGraw-Hill, 1969, © 1968. 280 pp.

87. Eissler, Kurt Robert. *The psychiatrist and the dying patient.* N.Y., International Universities Press; London, Bailey & Swinfen [distributor], 1955. 338 pp. Paperback ed.: N.Y., International Universities Press, 1969. 338 pp.

88. Glaser, Barney G., and Strauss, Anselm Leonard. *Awareness of dying.* [Based on the authors' field work conducted at six hospitals in the Bay area of San Francisco over a period of three years. With the collaboration of Jeanne Quint. With case illustrations. The first of a series of four monographs.] Chicago, Aldine, 1965. 305 pp. (Observations.) London, Weidenfeld & Nicolson, 1966. 305 pp.

89. Glaser, Barney G., and Strauss, Anselm Leonard. *Time for dying.* [Based on intensive field work at six hospitals in the Bay Area of San Francisco, supplemented with rapid field work at hospitals in Italy, Greece, and Scotland and on earlier observations made at hospitals in Asian countries. With case illustrations. The third of a series of four monographs resulting from a six-year research program.] Chicago, Aldine, 1968. 270 pp. (Observations.)

90. Verwoerdt, Adriaan. *Communication with the fatally ill.* [Based on the author's several years of clinical experience with fatally ill patients at Duke University Medical Center. With a bibliography.] Springfield, Ill., Thomas, 1966. 183 pp.

91. Kübler-Ross, Elisabeth. *On death and dying.* [Outgrowth of an interdisciplinary seminar on death and dying first held in 1965 by the author and four theology students of the Chicago Theological Seminary and developed in 1967 to an accredited course for the Medical School of the University of Chicago and the Chicago Theological Seminary. Based on interviews with terminally ill patients in the presence of students, held under the auspices of the Department of Psychiatry at the University of Chicago Billings Hospital. With extensive case illustrations and transcripts of the interviews. With a bibliography.] N.Y., Macmillan; London, Tavistock, 1969. 260 pp.

92. Mitchell, Marjorie Editha. *The child's attitude to death.* [Based in part on the author's investigations confined mainly to children of

primary school age in Britain. With excerpts from related studies and diverse autobiographical and other sources. With a bibliography.] London, Barrie & Rockliff in association with the Pemberton Publishing Co., 1966; N.Y., Schocken Books, 1967. 162 pp.

93. Kliman, Gilbert. *Psychological emergencies of childhood.* [Based on cases from the research and treatment files of the Center for Preventive Psychiatry, on the author's own practice, and on a study of healthy children's reactions to the death of a parent, conducted by the author and Ann Kliman at the Department of Child Psychiatry, Albert Einstein College of Medicine. Dedicated to the staff of the Center for Preventive Psychiatry and to the trustees of the Foundation for Research in Psychiatry, Marianne Kris, Mary O'Neil Hawkins, and Milton Berner. A volume in a series under the consultant editorship of Leopold Bellak. With extensive case reports, including one of a dying child in analysis at age four. With reviews of the psychoanalytic literature and a bibliography.] N.Y., Grune & Stratton; London, Heinemann Medical Books [distributor], 1968. 154 pp.

94. Hinde, Robert A. *Animal behaviour; a synthesis of ethology and comparative psychology.* [With reviews of the literature and an extensive bibliography.] N.Y., London, McGraw-Hill, 1966. 534 pp.

95. Sluckin, Władisław. *Imprinting and early learning.* [With a bibliography.] London, Methuen, 1964. 147 pp. (Methuen's manuals of modern psychology.) Chicago, Aldine, 1965. 147 pp.

96. Masserman, Jules Hymen. *The biodynamic roots of human behavior.* [With surveys of biological data from the ethological research literature and reports of animal experimental studies conducted by the author and his associates. With a bibliography.] Springfield, Ill., Thomas, 1968. 119 pp.

97. *Science and psychoanalysis.* Vol. 12: Animal and human; scientific proceedings [of the eleventh annual meeting] of the American Academy of Psychoanalysis, [held in Detroit, May 1967. Contributors: Joseph Barnett and others.] Edited by Jules H. Masserman. [With the presidential address: The medical model in psychoanalysis, by Ralph M. Crowley. With a paper: The psychoanalyst's role in community mental health centers, by Robert G. Heath and William H. Shelton. With reports and reviews of research and bibliographies.] N.Y., Grune & Stratton; London, Heinemann Medical Books [distributor], 1968. 277 pp.

98. Clemente, Carmine Domenic, and Lindsley, Donald Benjamin, eds. *Aggression and defense; neural mechanisms and social patterns.* Proceedings of the Fifth Conference on Brain Function [held in Pacific

Palisades] November [14th to 17th,] 1965; sponsored by the Brain Research Institute, University of California Los Angeles. Editors: Carmine D. Clemente and Donald B. Lindsley, [chairman. Participants: Jack D. Barchas and others. With a historical survey: Human aggression in psychiatric perspective, by Henry W. Brosin. With reports and reviews of research and bibliographies.] Berkeley, Univ. of California Pr.; London, Cambridge Univ. Pr. [distributor], 1968. 361 pp. (Brain function, vol. 5.) (UCLA forum in medical sciences, no. 7.)

99. Lorenz, Konrad. *On aggression.* Transl. [from the German, Das sogennante Böse; zur Naturgeschichte der Aggression, Wien, 1963] by Marjorie Kerr Wilson. [With a bibliography.] N.Y., Harcourt, Brace & World, 1966. 306 pp. (A Helen and Kurt Wolff book.) British ed.: Transl. by Marjorie Latzke. With a foreword by Sir Julian Huxley. London, Methuen, 1966. 273 pp. Paperback eds.: N.Y., Bantam Books, 1967. 306 pp. (Q3511.) London, Methuen, 1968. 273 pp. (University paperbacks.)

100. Storr, Anthony. *Human aggression.* [Dedicated to Konrad Lorenz. With bibliographies.] N.Y., Atheneum; London, Allen Lane, The Penguin Press, 1968. 127 pp.

101. Frank, Jerome David. *Sanity and survival; psychological aspects of war and peace.* [Pref. by J. William Fulbright. With a bibliography.] N.Y., Random House, 1967. 330 pp. Paperback ed.: N.Y., Vintage Books, a division of Random House, 1968. 330 pp. (A Vintage book, V-413.) London, Barrie & Rockliff, 1968. 330 pp.

102. American Anthropological Association. *War: the anthropology of armed conflict and aggression.* [Based on a symposium held on November 30, 1967, in Washington, D.C., during the Sixty-sixth Annual Meeting of the American Anthropological Association, Fred Eggan, chairman. Outgrowth of a petition signed by members of the American Anthropological Association at its annual meeting held at Pittsburgh, 1966. Contributors: Frank B. Livingstone and others.] Edited by Morton Fried, Marvin Harris, and Robert Murphy. [With a bibliography.] Garden City, N.Y., Published for the American Museum of Natural History by the Natural History Press, 1968. 262 pp.

103. Bowlby, John. *Attachment and loss.* [Outgrowth of the author's studies of maternal deprivation in collaboration with James Robertson and others, begun in the 1950's at the Tavistock Clinic and Tavistock Institute of Human Relations.] Vol. 1: *Attachment.* [With an appendix: The child's tie to his mother: review of the psychoanalytical literature, previously published, 1958. With reviews of the literature and a bibliography.] N.Y., Basic Books, 1969. 428 pp. London, Ho-

garth Press & Institute of Psycho-Analysis, 1969. 428 pp. (The International psycho-analytical library, no. 79.)

104. Mahler, Margaret Schoenberger. *On human symbiosis and the vicissitudes of individuation.* Vol. 1: *Infantile psychosis.* [Outgrowth of the author's experience in child psychoanalytic practice in Vienna before 1938, after 1940 at various institutions in New York, including the Children's Service of the New York State Psychiatric Institute, and on her four-year intensive study of symbiotic infantile psychosis, conducted with Manuel Furer in the 1950's mainly at the Masters Children's Center. Based in part on the author's papers previously published, 1951-1967.] In collaboration with Manuel Furer. [With extensive case reports and a bibliography.] N.Y., International Universities Press, 1968. London, Hogarth Press & Institute of Psycho-Analysis, 1969. 271 pp. (The International psycho-analytical library, no. 82.)

105. Furst, Sidney Selig, ed. *Psychic trauma.* [Contributors: Sidney S. Furst, Leo Rangell, Peter B. Neubauer, Phyllis Greenacre, Joseph Sandler, Albert J. Solnit and Marianne Kris, Robert Waelder, and Anna Freud. Dedicated to Herman Nunberg. Foreword by Peter B. Neubauer. With case histories, a survey of the psychoanalytic literature, and bibliographies.] N.Y., Basic Books; London, Harper & Row [distributor], 1967. 252 pp. (Monograph series sponsored by the Psychoanalytic Research and Development Fund, no. 1.)

106. Glover, Edward. *The birth of the ego; a nuclear hypothesis.* N.Y., International Universities Press; London, Allen & Unwin, 1968. 125 pp.

107. Arieti, Silvano. *The intrapsychic self; feeling, cognition, and creativity in health and mental illness.* [With a bibliography.] N.Y., Basic Books; London, Harper & Row [distributor], 1967. 487 pp.

108. Halloran, James Dermot. *Attitude formation and change.* [A survey of research on the socialization process and on attitude formation and change, mainly work done during the past fifteen years. Foreword by A. F. Noble. Appendix A: Moral development. Appendix B: Research methods, by Marie Jahoda. Appendix C: Television Research Committee. With a bibliography.] N.Y., Humanities Press [distributor]; Leicester, Leicester Univ. Pr., 1967. 167 pp. (Television Research Committee. Working paper no. 2.)

109. Dawson, Richard E., and Prewitt, Kenneth. *Political socialization: an analytic study.* [Series editors' foreword by Gabriel A. Almond, James S. Coleman, and Lucian W. Pye. With reviews of the literature.] Boston, Little, Brown, 1968, © 1969. 226 pp. (The Little, Brown series in comparative politics.)

110. Olesen, Virginia L., and Whittaker, Elvi W. *The silent dialogue; a study in the social psychology of professional socialization* [conducted at the University of California School of Nursing, San Francisco, Fred Davis, project director. Based largely on the authors' participant observation and fieldwork during the course of the study of 50 women, 1960-1963, and on questionnaires and semi-annual interviews. With excerpts from field notes and interviews.] San Francisco, Jossey-Bass, 1968. 312 pp. (The Jossey-Bass behavioral science series.)

111. Phillips, Leslie. *Human adaptation and its failures.* [A report of work in progress in a number of long-term research projects carried out by the author and his co-workers over fifteen years, partly under the auspices of the Worcester State Hospital. With reviews of the literature and bibliographies.] N.Y., London, Academic Press, 1968. 271 pp. (Personality and psychopathology; a series of monographs, texts, and treatises, 3.)

112. Pringle, Mia Lilly Kellmer. *Social learning and its measurement.* [Report of a British study of Doll's Vineland Social Maturity Scale. Based on the author's study of 250 children, six to eight years old, using tests, interviews, and teachers' ratings. Foreword by C. A. Mace. With a chapter: Discrepancies between intelligence and social competence, written in collaboration with W. D. Wall. With extensive case material, reviews of American and British studies, and a bibliography.] London, Longmans, 1966; N.Y., Humanities Press, 1967. 100 pp. (Education today.)

113. Vernon, Philip Ewart. *Intelligence and cultural environment.* [Final report to the Association for the Aid of Crippled Children, New York, on the author's cross-cultural studies carried out under its auspices. Based largely on a battery of tests given by the author and Dorothy Vernon to 375 boys aged around eleven years in England, Scotland, Jamaica, Uganda, and Eskimos and Indians in Canada. With extensive reviews of the literature and of studies involving testing in Britain, the United States, and non-Western cultures, and a bibliography.] N.Y., Barnes & Noble [distributor]; London, Methuen, 1969. 264 pp. (Methuen's manuals of modern psychology.)

114. Green, Richard, and Money, John, eds. *Transsexualism and sex reassignment.* [Contributors: Harry Benjamin and others. Dedicated to Harry Benjamin. Foreword by Reed Erickson. With extensive case material, reports of research, and a bibliography.] Baltimore, London, Johns Hopkins Press, 1969. 512 pp.

115. Koch, Helen Lois. *Twins and twin relations.* [Report of a study of 96 pairs of twins, fifty-nine to eighty-six months in age, chil-

dren of white, urban or suburban families in the Chicago area. Based in part on interviews with the children, their mothers and teachers, on tests and teachers' ratings. With reviews of the literature and a bibliography.] Chicago, London, Univ. of Chicago Pr., 1966. 302 pp.

116. Scheinfeld, Amram. *Twins and supertwins.* With special editing by Arthur Falek and others herein mentioned. The first comprehensive account of the lives of the multiple-born from conception through maturity—their type differences, health factors, psychological traits, social relationships, unique experiences, and special problems—as revealed by scientists, by parents of twins, and by twins themselves. [Based on information obtained by the author from and/or regarding more than 1,100 individual members of twin pairs, partly with the co-operation of Mothers of Twins clubs.] Illustrated by the author. [Appendix 1: Trailblazers in twin study. Appendix 2: Organizations and clinics. With a bibliography.] Philadelphia, Lippincott, 1967; London, Chatto & Windus, 1968. 292 pp.

117. De Hirsch, Katrina, Jansky, Jeannette Jefferson, and Langford, William S. *Predicting reading failure; a preliminary study of reading, writing, and spelling disabilities in preschool children.* [Outgrowth of the authors' experience with children at the Pediatric Language Disorder Clinic, Babies Hospital, Columbia-Presbyterian Medical Center, New York. A study of 30 boys and 23 girls, 5 years 2 months to 6 years 6 months old over a period of 2½ years, and of 53 prematurely born children. Foreword by Lauretta Bender. With a description of the 37 kindergarten tests used and with bibliographies.] N.Y., London, Harper & Row, 1966. 144 pp.

118. Wyatt, Gertrud L. *Language learning and communication disorders in children.* [Based on the author's clinical observations of children's language behavior made partly in Central European and partly in North American settings, and on a series of research studies carried out during the last ten years by the author and her collaborators at the Wellesley Public Schools, Wellesley, Massachusetts. Foreword by Dorothea McCarthy. With extensive case histories, including the case of the language development of the author's own child observed from birth to adolescence. With a survey of programs of compensatory education for young children. With a verbatim transcript of a tape-recorded interview between a therapist and the mother of a stuttering child. With reviews of the literature and a bibliography.] N.Y., Free Press; London, Collier-Macmillan, 1969. 372 pp.

119. Bettelheim, Bruno. *The children of the dream.* [Based largely on the author's study of communal rearing in the Israeli kibbutz Atid,

*pseud.*, during seven weeks in 1964, using tape-recorded interviews with several hundred persons and other materials. Dedicated to Jeremiah Kaplan. With case material and a bibliography.] N.Y., Macmillan; London, Thames & Hudson, 1969. 363 pp. Paperback ed. with subtitle: *Communal child-rearing and American education.* N.Y., Avon Books, 1970. 380 pp. (Avon, J101.)

120. Davis, Carroll. *Room to grow; a study of parent-child relationships.* [Based on the author's analysis, made with Dorothy A. Millichamp and Pearl Karal, of data collected at the Institute of Child Study, Toronto, over a period of thirty years, obtained from the sixth year to late adolescence for children attending the Institute's nursery school between 1926 and 1945. Foreword by Mary D. Salter Ainsworth. With the stories of seven children and a bibliography.] Toronto, Univ. of Toronto Pr., 1966; London, Univ. of London Pr., 1967. 214 pp.

121. Newson, John, and Newson, Elizabeth. *Four years old in an urban community.* [Report of the second phase in a long-term project, a study of 700 children in Nottingham, England, 275 of whom had been included in the authors' study of mothers and their year-old babies published as *Infant care in an urban community,* N.Y., London, 1963. Based on interviews with the mothers. With excerpts from the interviews and the transcript of the same interview with the investigators' four-year-old daughter about her experiences in bringing up an imaginary four-year-old child. With a bibliography.] Chicago, Aldine; London, Allen & Unwin, 1968. 570 pp.

122. Ferguson, Thomas. *Children in care–and after.* [A study of 110 boys and 95 girls who had been in the care of the Children's Department in Glasgow after they had left care at the age of eighteen attained 1961-1963. With case illustrations and a historical survey of the boarding-out system in Glasgow.] N.Y., London, Published for the Nuffield Foundation by Oxford Univ. Pr., 1966. 139 pp.

123. McWhinnie, Alexina Mary. *Adopted children: how they grow up; a study of their adjustment as adults.* [Based on interviews conducted 1954-1956 with 58 adults, aged eighteen to sixty years, who had been adopted as children. A shortened version of the author's Ph.D. thesis, University of Edinburgh, 1960.] Foreword by Eileen Younghusband. [With a historical review of adoption legislation in Great Britain. With a review of previous relevant research studies, case histories, and a bibliography.] N.Y., Humanities Press; London, Routledge & Paul, 1967. 302 pp. (International library of sociology and social reconstruction.)

124. Robins, Lee Nelken. *Deviant children grown up; a sociological*

*and psychiatric study of sociopathic personality.* [The product of ten years of research into the adult status of 524 child guidance clinic patients, compared with a control group of 100 nonpatient school children. Based on interviews and records obtained in a follow-up study after thirty years. With an introd. by Leon Eisenberg. With a list of 17 previous publications from this study, 1958-1966, and a bibliography.] Baltimore, Williams & Wilkins; Edinburgh, Livingstone, 1966. 351 pp.

125. Pringle, Mia Lilly Kellmer. *Adoption, facts and fallacies; a review of research in the United States, Canada and Great Britain between 1948 and 1965.* [A study begun in 1965 as part of a larger enquiry sponsored by the Home Office.] With the assistance of Micheline Dewdney, Eileen Crellin, and Rosemary Dinnage. [Foreword by J. B. Howard. With abstracts of completed research projects, an annotated bibliography, and annotated lists of ongoing research projects.] N.Y., Humanities Press [distributor]; London, Longmans in association with the National Bureau for Co-operation in Child Care, 1967. 251 pp. (Studies in child development.)

126. Helfer, Ray E., and Kempe, C. Henry, eds. *The battered child.* [Contributors: Jack G. Collins, Elizabeth L. Davoren, David G. Gil, Ray E. Helfer, C. Henry Kempe, Monrad G. Paulsen, Carl B. Pollock, Frederic N. Silverman, Brandt F. Steele, and James Tutthill Weston.] With a foreword by Katherine B. Oettinger. [With a history of child abuse and infanticide, by Samuel X. Radbill. With case material and reports and reviews of research. Appendixes: A. California Pilot Study. B. A summary of neglect and traumatic cases. C. A summary of child abuse legislation. With bibliographies.] Chicago, London, Univ. of Chicago Pr., 1968. 268 pp.

127. Goldstein, Bernard. *Low income youth in urban areas;* a critical review of the literature, [primarily material published 1950-1966.] With the assistance of Barbara Steinberg and Harry C. Bredemeier. [Dedicated to Louis Wirth. With annotated references.] N.Y., London, Holt, Rinehart & Winston, 1967. 280 pp.

128. Chilman, Catherine S. *Growing up poor; an over-view and analysis of child-rearing and family life patterns associated with poverty. Implications for the mental health, educational achievement, social behavior, family stability of very poor parents and their children. Suggestions for action programs. Guidelines to further research.* [Based upon a review of recent studies. Prefatory note by Ellen Winston. Foreword by Genevieve W. Carter. With a bibliography.] Washington, U.S. Dept. of Health, Education, and Welfare, Welfare Administration,

Division of Research, 1966. 117 pp. (U.S. Welfare Administration. Publication no. 13.)

129. Coles, Robert. *Children of crisis; a study of courage and fear.* [An account of a New England psychiatrist's study begun in the late 1950's and carried out over a period of eight years, based largely on interviews with Negro children and adults in various parts of the South and on participant-observation. With extensive case material, edited extracts from interviews, and reproductions of children's drawings.] Boston, Little, Brown, 1967. 401 pp. (An Atlantic Monthly press book.) London, Faber & Faber, 1968. 401 pp. Paperback ed.: With illustrations. N.Y., Dell, 1968. 401 pp. (A Delta book, 1235.)

130. Pavenstedt, Eleanor, ed. *The drifters: children of disorganized lower-class families,* by Charles A. Malone, Eleanor Pavenstedt, Ilse Mattick, Louise S. Bandler, Maurice R. Stein, and Norbett L. Mintz. [Based on the North Point Family Project, 1955-1959, undertaken under the auspices of the Boston University-Boston City Hospital Guidance Clinic in the Department of Child Psychiatry of the Division of Psychiatry, Boston University School of Medicine and on the North Point Demonstration Project, 1960-1965, representing intensive work with thirteen families and their 45 pre-school children.] Foreword by Bernard Bandler. [With a survey of remedial programs for multiproblem families and their preschool children. With bibliographies.] Boston, Little, Brown; London, Churchill, 1967. 345 pp.

131. Deutsch, Martin, and associates. *The disadvantaged child; selected papers of Martin Deutsch and associates* [Richard D. Bloom, Bert R. Brown, Cynthia P. Deutsch, Leo S. Goldstein, Vera P. John, Phyllis A. Katz, Alma Levinson, Estelle Cherry Peisach, and Martin Whiteman. Partly previously published, 1960-1966. With reports of research and bibliographies.] N.Y., Basic Books; London, Harper & Row [distributor], 1967. 400 pp.

132. International Conference on Malnutrition, Learning, and Behavior, Massachusetts Institute of Technology, 1967. *Malnutrition, learning, and behavior; proceedings of an international conference co-sponsored by the Nutrition Foundation, Inc., and the Massachusetts Institute of Technology, held at Cambridge, Massachusetts, March 1 to 3, 1967.* [Planning Committee: David Coursin, Gilbert Forbes, Paul B. Pearson, chairman, Nevin S. Scrimshaw, Horace L. Sipple, and Dwain N. Walcher. Participants: Howard W. Johnson and others.] Edited [and with a running comment] by Nevin S. Scrimshaw and John E. Gordon. [With reports and reviews of research and bibliographies.] Cambridge, London, M.I.T. Press, 1968. 566 pp.

133. Piaget, Jean. *Six psychological studies* [previously published or presented, 1940-1964]. With an introd., notes, and glossary by David Elkind. Translation from the French [Six études de psychologie, Genève, 1964] by Anita Tenzer. Translation edited by David Elkind. [With a bibliography.] N.Y., Random House, 1967; London, Univ. of London Pr., 1969. 169 pp. Paperback ed.: N.Y., Vintage Books, a division of Random House, 1968. 169 pp. (A Vintage book, V-462.)

134. Piaget, Jean, and Inhelder, Bärbel. *The psychology of the child.* [A synthesis of the authors' published studies.] Translated from the French [ La psychologie de l'enfant, Paris, 1966] by Helen Weaver. [With a bibliography.] N.Y., Basic Books; London, Routledge & Paul, 1969. 173 pp.

135. Phillips, John Lawrence, Jr. *The origins of intellect: Piaget's theory.* [With case illustrations and a bibliography.] San Francisco; Folkstone, Kent, Freeman, 1969. 149 pp. (A series of books in psychology.)

136. Erikson, Erik Homburger. *Young man Luther; a study in psychoanalysis and history.* N.Y., Norton, 1958. 288 pp. (Austen Riggs monograph no. 4.) London, Faber & Faber, 1959. 280 pp. Paperback ed.: N.Y., Norton, 1962. 288 pp. (The Norton library, N170.)

137. Erikson, Erik Homburger. *Identity: youth and crisis.* [Dedicated to the memory of Robert P. Knight and David Rapaport. A successor to the author's *Childhood and society,* N.Y., 1950, and a companion volume to his *Young man Luther,* N.Y., 1958. With a list of the author's writings on which this book is based, 1946-1967, and a bibliography.] N.Y., Norton, London, Faber & Faber, 1968. 336 pp.

138. Evans, Richard Isadore. *Dialogue with Erik Erikson.* [Based on edited transcripts of 16-mm. sound films and additional audio-taped dialogues. With a bibliography and a list of Erikson's publications, 1930-1966.] N.Y., London, Harper & Row, 1967. 142 pp. (Dialogues with notable contributors to personality theory, vol. 3.)

139. Sears, Robert Richardson, Rau, Lucy, and Alpert, Richard. *Identification and child rearing.* [Report of a study begun in 1956 at the Laboratory of Human Development, Stanford University. Based on research conducted with 21 boys and 19 girls at the Stanford Village Nursery School, 1958. With a bibliography.] Stanford, Calif., Stanford Univ. Pr., 1965; London, Tavistock, 1966. 383 pp. (Stanford studies in psychology, 4.)

140. Freud, Anna. *The writings of Anna Freud.* Vol. 4: *Indications for child analysis and other papers, 1945-1956.* [Outgrowth of the author's extension of activities from private practice to clinic practice

with children at the Hampstead Child-Therapy Course and Clinic, London. With an abstract of the author's Freud anniversary lecture: *Psychoanalysis and education,* presented at the New York Academy of Medicine, May 5, 1954, reprinted from the Psychoanalytic Study of the Child, vol. 9, 1954. With two previously unpublished papers and two papers previously published in German, appearing here in English for the first time. With case material and a bibliography.] N.Y., International Universities Press, 1968. 690 pp. London, Hogarth Press & Institute of Psycho-Analysis, 1969. 690 pp. (The International psychoanalytical library, no. 80.)

141. Marrow, Alfred Jay. *The practical theorist; the life and work of Kurt Lewin.* [Based in part on the author's association with Kurt Lewin from 1934 to 1947 and on the reflections of Lewin's former students, colleagues, and associates, Donald K. Adams and others, obtained in writing or in expanded conversations. Dedicated to the Research Center for Group Dynamics (Massachusetts Institute of Technology, 1945-1947; University of Michigan, 1947- ). With a list of the recipients of the Kurt Lewin award of the Society for the Psychological Study of Social Issues and their annual Kurt Lewin memorial lectures, 1948-1969. With a bibliography of the works of Kurt Lewin, 1917-1960. With summaries of the Berlin experiments, mostly doctoral dissertations, reported in the Psychologische Forschung, 1927-1934. With a list of the members of the Topology Group, 1935. With an annotated list of the Iowa studies, 1937-1944. With a classified, annotated list of the publications based on the action-research projects of the Commission on Community Interrelations for the American Jewish Congress, 1945-1953. With a list of Research Center for Group Dynamics publications, 1945-1950.] N.Y., Basic Books; London, Harper & Row [distributor], 1969. 290 pp.

142. Parfit, Jessie, ed. *The community's children; long-term substitute care: a guide for the intelligent layman.* [Outgrowth of the discussions of a working party set up in 1964 by the Association of Child Psychology and Psychiatry in collaboration with the National Bureau for Co-operation in Child Care, to consider the "Management and Treatment of Emotional Problems of Children in Care," M. L. Kellmer Pringle, convener and chairman. Contributors: Kenneth Brill, Joan D. Cooper, Morris Horovitch, Alan A. Jacka, J. M. Lomax-Simpson, Lydia Mundy, M. L. Kellmer Pringle, Margery H. Taylor, and D. W. Winnicott. Foreword by D. W. Winnicott. With case examples. With an appendix: Relevant laws and with a bibliography.] N.Y., Humanities Press in association with the National Bureau for Co-operation

in Child Care (England); London, Longmans in association with the National Bureau for Co-operation in Child Care, 1967. 108 pp. (Studies in child development.)

143. Gooch, Stan, and Pringle, Mia Lilly Kellmer. *Four years on; a follow-up study at school leaving age of children formerly attending a traditional and a progressive junior school.* [Study of a follow-up sample of 81 children aged fifteen years in 1964, scoring in the lower 60 percent of scores on the Neale Analysis of Reading Ability at the age of eleven, from an original population of 262 boys and girls intensively studied between the ages of seven and eleven years (1956-1960) at Townsend, *pseud.*, and Parkside, *pseud.*, schools. Based on standardized tests, projective material, and questionnaires. Foreword by Sir George Haynes. With excerpts from children's responses, reviews of related studies, and bibliographies.] N.Y., Humanities Press [distributor]; London, Published in association with the National Bureau for Co-operation in Child Care by Longmans, 1966. 167 pp. (Studies in child development.)

144. Humphrey, Michael. *The hostage seekers; a study of childless and adopting couples.* [Based on interviews conducted in 1966 with 40 adoptive and 40 childless women drawn from 216 respondents to a questionnaire sent in 1965 to 320 women who had attended a hospital infertility clinic during the years 1955 to 1964. Foreword by D. A. Pond. With case material and a bibliography.] N.Y., Humanities Press [distributor]; London, Longmans in association with the National Bureau for Co-operation in Child Care, 1969. 162 pp. (Studies in child development.)

145. Des Lauriers, Austin Mark, and Carlson, Carole Ferne. *Your child is asleep; early infantile autism: etiology, treatment, parental influences.* [Reports of the authors' research and treatment program with five autistic children between the ages of two and six years and their parents, carried out on an out-patient basis. Outgrowth of a broad study of the Parental Influences on Early Ego Development in the Child. With the clinical report by the mother of one of the children. With a review of the literature and a bibliography.] Homewood, Ill., Dorsey Press, 1969. 403 pp. (The Dorsey series in psychology.)

146. Liebow, Elliot. *Tally's corner; a study of Negro streetcorner men.* [Based largely on data collected 1962-1963 for the research project, "Child Rearing Practices among Low-Income Families in the District of Columbia," carried out by the Health and Welfare Council of the National Capital Area.] With a foreword by Hylan Lewis. [Revision of the author's Ph.D. thesis in anthropology, Catholic University

of America. With a bibliography.] Boston, Little, Brown, 1967. 260 pp. British ed. with title: *Tally's corner,* Washington, D.C. London, Routledge & Paul, 1967. 260 pp.

147. Hirsch, Jerry, ed. *Behavior-genetic analysis.* [Based on two conferences on heredity and behavior held in August 1961 and in August 1962 at the Center for Advanced Study in the Behavioral Sciences, Stanford, California. Participants: Gordon Allen and others. Contributors: Ernst W. Caspari and others. Dedicated to Robert Choate Tryon. Foreword by Theodosius Dobzhansky. With reviews of the literature and an extensive bibliography.] N.Y., London, McGraw-Hill, 1967. 522 pp. (McGraw-Hill series in psychology.)

# ESSAY 14

## *The Emerging Field of Sociobibliography: Reassessment and Reorientation of Access to Knowledge in the Social Sciences*[1]

Originally published as Editorial in *Mental Health Book Review Index,* vol. 17, (whole no. 22), 1972.

Access to knowledge in the social sciences requires a new understanding of the nature of scientific literature. Bibliography, as a tradition-bound technique, was not prepared for the advent of the computer. Therefore, although technological innovations of the past two decades were applied to bibliographic systems, these systems themselves remained conventional. In order to bring about the necessary intellectual innovations, we need a scientific approach to bibliography. The term "sociobibliography" indicates such a new approach. This emerging field focuses on issues of common concern to the social sciences and bibliography, and it does so by merging methods of social and bibliographic research.

Traditionally, the purpose of bibliography has been to provide references to publications, and scientific interest has centered on the substance of the publications. In sociobibliography, bibliographic data are investigated for a variety of scientific purposes independent of users' needs to consult the publications.

One such purpose, for example, would be to explore the factors that have made much of our bibliographic organization conceptually obsolete. When bibliographic systems communicate ideas in a form that is no longer in keeping with current scientific and social thought, this not only means a decline of scholarship, it also constitutes a social issue.

To make terminological changes in specific instances is not sufficient. A sociobibliographic study would be concerned with the principle of obsolescence in bibliographic organization in relation to changing scientific and ideological trends and would seek ways of avoiding the underlying dilemma.

In the process of extending scientific theory and research to a long-neglected problem area, sociobibliography will also have to develop the necessary competence and resources.

In the application of sociobibliography to problems of the literature of the social sciences, the formation of this literature becomes apparent as a result of the work of the scientific community, whose members contribute to it not only as authors but as editors and in various other roles as well.

First, however, the question of what the social sciences are should be considered. Definitions of the social sciences can be structural or functional. In libraries, in bibliographic systems, and in other practical contexts, the social sciences are usually defined in structural terms as a group of disciplines such as political science, sociology, economics, and anthropology. The actual arrangement of library collections and bibliographic services reflects also various older layers of structural organization. The literature in the fields of history and linguistics, for example, is now divided between the social sciences and the humanities. In some fields now included in the social sciences, such as law and education, the literature is still kept separate on the basis of professional specialization. In the health sciences, bibliographic organization remains in the domain of the biomedical sciences. This poses serious problems of access to knowledge increasingly needed also in the social sciences.

The functional type of definition is used, for example, by Norman W. Storer and Talcott Parsons, who state that the social sciences are concerned with social action. They describe social action as behavior in the physical world—the domain of the natural sciences—which is guided by culture—the domain of the humanities ("The Disciplines as a Differentiating Force." In Montgomery, Edward B., ed. *The Foundations of Access to Knowledge; a Symposium.* Syracuse, New York, Syracuse University, 1968; pp. 101-121; p. 111.) A functional definition of the social sciences need not be as general as that, however. It can be made specific and concrete by considering the important social issues of our time. The issues of population growth, hunger and malnutrition, and peace research illustrate the need for integrated knowledge drawn from diverse fields, many of which lie outside of the social sciences as now organized. The problem posed to sociobibliography is twofold: (1) the prevailing bibliographic organization of the literature of the social sciences does not provide a reasonably complete, much less an integrative access to knowledge on most of the significant issues of our time; and (2) there are no bibliographic methods and systems that can reflect progress in the social sciences as a still evolving and expanding major area of knowledge.

## ACCESS TO KNOWLEDGE IN THE SOCIAL SCIENCES

The difference between information and knowledge is not absolute but involves various stages in a process that transforms information into knowledge. As the term "scientific information" correctly implies, many information specialists have focused their interest on the stages that are closest to information, especially journal articles, information exchanges prior to publication, and even the storing of raw data. We are concerned with the later stages of the process that are closer to knowledge and ask: How does information move forward through the channels of the literature? And how does it become consolidated and integrated into knowledge? We therefore examine the formation of the literature of the social sciences in three consecutive stages: the journal literature, the monographic literature, and the book review literature.

## THE JOURNAL LITERATURE

The journal literature developed with the rise of modern science in the last third of the 17th century. The organization of journals involved an editor and editorial board, the use of referees, and often sponsorship by a learned society. As the sociologists Harriet Zuckerman and Robert K. Merton have shown in a recent study ("Patterns of Evaluation in Science: Institutionalization, Structure and Functions of the Referee System." *Minerva,* 1971, 9, 66-100), these patterns were set almost from the start in the earliest journals. At that time it was necessary to induce scientists to share their work through publication, in exchange for recognition of their intellectual property rights and the critical review by their peers. Competent appraisal of papers by a journal's editor and referees has remained the basis for scientific standards and prestige in the journal literature.

When the scientific community developed a system that led to the formation of the scientific journal literature, the work done by scientists in the various roles was not acknowledged in the same way. A scientist received full public recognition for a paper published in a journal. What he contributed to a journal in his capacity as editor or referee was not identified, however. With the passage of three centuries, the burden of sifting and editing manuscripts for journal publication has increased enormously. In various groups of current journals, the rejection rate for manuscripts has been shown to range from 30 to 90% (Zuckerman & Merton, *op. cit.*, pp. 75-80). Nonetheless, the shared effort and involvement of the scientific community is still not easily apparent from a system that, with respect to explicit credit, places the chief emphasis on authorship. That one-sided emphasis has been magnified in the indexing and abstracting systems, which are also centered on the authors of articles and the titles of journals. Although the journal editor wields the power of acceptance and rejection, makes the policy decisions, and actually gives direction and form to the progress of knowledge, the significance of his function is not shown in the bibliographic record.

The interplay between editorship and authorship and its neglect in bibliography can be illustrated from the life and work of Freud. His early psychoanalytic papers of the 1890's were accepted by editors of journals in established fields, and Freud himself commented on the fact that this could not have been taken for granted. Even now, editorial support for innovative ideas must come from existing journals until new channels for the innovations are created. Sociobibliography can throw new light on the question of how the scientific community adapts to and absorbs new knowledge.

Repeatedly and over several decades, Freud was also actively involved in editorship, but the salient facts and writings relating to Freud's role as editor went unnoticed until the second half of the century. They still cannot easily be reconstructed from the representative psychoanalytic bibliographies, and not at all from more general bibliographic sources.

The lack of scholarly attention paid to editorial functions extends to the journal editorial. It has remained outside of the bibliographic record, and it also has not been studied as a social invention of the scientific community. The findings of such a study could change the narrow concept of scientific literature as serving only the purpose of reporting facts. In addition, it would be possible to use journal editorials as a means for tracing and projecting major scientific and cultural trends, since they are often directed to that border area between science and society where issues of scientific research converge with issues of social policy and social action.

Since little is known about the basic facts regarding editorship, changes that have occurred with respect to editorial and reviewing functions have also been hardly noticed. A significant trend, for example, has led from anonymity to identification of those who assess, consolidate, and organize contributions to the literature and eventually to knowledge. Over a period of time that has yet to be established, identification appears to have progressed from editor-in-chief and members of the editorial board to book reviewers and book review editors, and, very recently, to referees. A growing number of journals now list once a year the names of those who have reviewed manuscripts, a development that opens entirely new perspectives to sociobibliography. For a thorough reassessment of the question of what bibliographic records of the journal literature should retain and what they should omit, it will be necessary to develop, from the original sources, a sociobibliographic guide to the names, policies, concepts, and issues relating to editorial functions and writings.

## THE MONOGRAPHIC LITERATURE

During the three hundred years since the invention of the scientific journal various other types of scientific literature have developed which, together, form the scientific monographic literature. This literature, too, is characterized by the involvement of the scientific community, as is suggested in a survey of the following seven groups:

1. *Journal supplements and special issues.* Special journal issues, usually devoted to a special topic or to independent publica-

tions such as congress proceedings, are often treated also as books.

2. *Collections of reprinted articles.* These involve a new process of selection and integration. The selection is usually centered on papers previously published by one author or about a particular topic.
3. *Works based on previous publications.* The books in this group include textbooks and many other works that attempt to integrate and to present in a new form previously reported theories and research.
4. *Comprehensive reviews and handbooks.* These works result from a comprehensive evaluation and integration of the substance of previous publications and are intended to minimize the need for other specialists to examine all the original sources on a subject cited indiscriminately in information services.
5. *Conference proceedings and other original presentations.* This group also comprises collections of invited papers, research studies, including technical reports, not previously published in journals, and independently written books and treatises. The involvement of the scientific community is provided by the organizers and participants of conferences and symposia, by editors, and by critical review before and after publication.
6. *Monographic series.* In series that bring books or pamphlets together under a unifying theme, the scientific community is represented by the series editor and often by scholarly auspices. Monographic series vary greatly in quality, however, ranging from integrative scholarly contributions to promotional devices of publishers.
7. *Invited lectures and festschriften.* These two types of monographic literature developed at different periods outside of the systems of organized science and reemphasize the individual scholar's autonomy. Their quality rests on an intrinsic honor system rather than on the constraints of the scientific community exerted from outside. These publications are often the channels for the communication of novel and germinal ideas and the expression of a scholar's concern with values.

An analysis of these groups suggests that the majority of scientific books are anchored in the operations of the scientific community. The monographs in the first four groups are variants of the journal literature, or they assess and reorganize it. The original presentations in the fifth group are selected and organized in comparable ways. The last two groups mark new beginnings toward generating, integrating, and organizing knowledge.

The various stages of evaluated and consolidated knowledge represented in this monographic literature remain hidden, when these works are absorbed either into the traditional catalogs of books or into the primarily journal-based indexing and abstracting services. In order to devise more distinctive bibliographic systems, it will be necessary to undertake a critical study of the various types and to demonstrate, through new bibliographic methods, the involvement of the scientific community and the diversity of formative processes in scientific literature.

## THE BOOK REVIEW LITERATURE

The third major stage in the formation of scientific literature is reached in the book review literature. It results from a series of processes involving selection and evaluation by specialists and is particularly significant in the area of the social and behavioral sciences. The book review literature, as another and relatively recent innovation of the scientific community, becomes visible, however, only through a sociobibliographic innovation. This is being shown in a pilot study, the *Mental Health Book Review Index,* which integrates book review citations from a large, multidisciplinary group of journals in the behavioral sciences. A further selection for a bibliographic presentation of books and book reviews is made when it appears that a certain level of authoritative, cross-disciplinary evaluation has been attained. Many basic data for research into the problems of access to knowledge might be provided by developing such a program for the broader area of the social sciences.

## THE PRINCIPLES OF SOCIOBIBLIOGRAPHY

The reorientation that results in sociobibliography as a new discipline is reflected in its basic principles, which are derived from important scientific and social perspectives of our time.

The first principle concerns adopting a forward direction in dealing with the literature of the social sciences. In addition to its new approaches to the history of ideas and social history, sociobibliography will direct its main pioneer effort to the detection and bibliographic presentation of novel concepts, incipient trends, and germinal ideas, and will attempt to forecast as well as to trace the direction in which the social sciences are moving.

The second principle of sociobibliography relates to the concept of optimal growth. A premise of information systems has been that the uncontrollable exponential growth in the number of publications can be managed only through the mass processing of unselected publications by computer. Sociobibliography starts from the premise that the scientific community exerts its own controls on growth. It recognizes that the processes of selection and rejection continuously performed by specialists offer an operational basis for avoiding malignant growth.

The third principle is an extension of the other two. It concerns the conservation of intellectual resources through the recycling and reuse of the competent work already done throughout the stages that lead to the formation of the scientific literature. Many information specialists have linked the advantage of the computer to the prospect of minimizing an intervening application of the human intellect and have used computers to process data directly available from publications. Sociobibliography first strengthens the application of the human intellect. To the competence of specialists that has already been invested in the scientific literature it adds an advanced bibliographic competence. The data generated from these successive processes of assessment, integration, and reorganization of knowledge could then be considered for computer applications.

Our purpose is not to offer solutions to the problem of access to knowledge in the social sciences, but rather to present a new basis for identifying and clarifying the problem itself. In the past, scientific literature has been considered from the standpoint of its substance and its use. It has, however, not only substance but also form, and it is not only used but also created. By studying all four dimensions of the literature of the social sciences, sociobibliography will seek to gain and to provide access to knowledge not only in the area of the social sciences, but also about the social sciences, about their nature, their literature, and the scientific community identified with them.

## NOTE

1. Summary of a paper prepared by Dr. Bry, as adjunct professor in the Library Science Department, for the Conference on Access to Knowledge and Information in the Social Sciences and Humanities: Problems and Implications, April 5–6, 1972, New York City, Library Science Department, Queens College of the City University of New York.

# Index

## ABOUT THE EDITORS

**Lois Afflerbach** is an assistant professor in the library department at Queens College, New York City. She specializes in sociology bibliography and reference, and her previous works include the *Mental Health Book Review Index,* which she coedited with Dr. Bry.

**Marga Franck** is manager of the Ludwig Vogelstein Foundation, Inc., in New York City. For many years, she was with the H. W. Wilson Company, where she edited the second supplement to the *Union List of Serials* and the *Bibliographic Index.* She has also written articles for library journals and other periodicals.

www.ingramcontent.com/pod-product-compliance
Ingram Content Group UK Ltd.
Pitfield, Milton Keynes, MK11 3LW, UK
UKHW020206290926
15470UKWH00001B/24

9 780837 1928